DASH DIET

COOKBOOK FOR TWO

A BEGINNER'S BOOK TO DISCOVER THE BEST WEIGHT LOSS
SOLUTION ON THE MARKET FOR DIABETICS AND NOT,
INCLUDING A 21-DAY MEAL PLAN

TABLE OF CONTENTS

INTRODUCTION

The DASH eating plan emphasizes on vegetables, fruits, whole grains, and low-fat dairy products, making it an ideal plan for anyone looking to gain health through lowered blood pressure and a healthier heart. The DASH plan has no specialized recipes or food plans. Daily caloric intake depends on a person's activity level and age. People who need to lose weight would naturally eat fewer calories.

When filling the plate for a meal, the food must be attractive, as well as tasty and nutritious. A wide variety of foods will make this plan much more enjoyable. Try to make choices that will offer a range of colors and textures. Remember that dessert is not off-limits but should be based around healthy choices that include fresh fruit.

The DASH diet's primary focus is on grains, vegetables, and fruits because these foods are higher fiber foods and will make you feel full longer. Whole grains should be consumed six to eight times daily, vegetables four to six servings daily, and fruit four to five servings daily. Low-fat dairy is an essential part of the diet and should be eaten two to three times daily. Also, there should be six or fewer servings daily of fish, poultry, and lean meat.

The DASH diet leans heavily on vegetables, fruits, and whole grains. Fish and lean poultry are served moderately. Whole wheat flour is used instead of white flour. DASH as a diet plan promotes low-fat dairy, lean meat, fruits, and vegetables. It is a mix of the old world and new world eating plans. It has been designed to follow past-diet principles to help eliminate new world health problems.

The carbohydrates are mainly made of plant fiber that the body does not easily digest and cannot turn into stored fat. The plan is rich in good fats that make food taste good and help us feel fuller for a more extended period. Proteins are not forbidden but are geared more toward plant-based protein and not so much meat consumption.

The DASH diet focuses on long-term healthy eating habits. The diet doesn't force you to starve or battle constant cravings. Instead, it focuses on understanding food groups, controlling portion sizes, and ensuring you get the optimal levels of potassium, calcium, magnesium, fiber, and protein.

The diet focuses on certain food groups for specific reasons: fruits and vegetables provide you the magnesium and potassium your body needs, and low-fat dairy products calcium. Every food you eat should have a purpose, and that's the most important principle of the DASH diet: eat well, so you feel well.

CHAPTER 1.

WHAT CAN I EAT?

Suitable and Unsuitable Foods

A DASH diet can be easily integrated into daily life simply because it uses available foods in conventional grocery stores. Depending on your calorie requirement, this is a guide to the amount of individual foods that can be consumed.

Allowed

Plenty of fresh vegetables, especially lots of greens (almost without restriction)

Fresh fruit

Lean meats, especially white meat (chicken, turkey)

Whole grain / whole grain products

Fish

Protein-rich foods

Foods with unsaturated and healthy fats, such as nuts and avocados

Healthy oils with an optimal Omega3 / 6 ratio, such as olive oil and coconut oil

Lean dairy products

Nuts, seeds, legumes

In Small Amounts

Alcohol

Coffee

Animal fats, especially red meat

Sweets and sugar

Avoid As Much as Possible

Ready meals and canned food

Sausages

Bakery products

Hydrogenated vegetable fats such as palm fat

Sunflower oil (poor omega3 / 6 ratio)

Pickled and smoked foods

DASH Diet Shopping List

The glycemic index (GI) differentiates foods according to their effect on blood sugar levels. The lower the GI, the more the DASH diet recommends this food.

Low GI Vegetables (1st Choice) (3 Servings/Day)
Artichokes
Aborigine
Avocados
Cauliflower
Broccoli
Green beans
Kale
Cucumbers
Cabbage
Pumpkin (summer squash)
Swiss chard
Paprika
Mushrooms
Radish
Brussels sprouts
Arugula
Salad (the darker the green, better)
Celery
Mustard seeds
Asparagus
Spinach
Sprouts
Zucchini
Sweet peas
Onions

Medium GI Vegetables (2nd Choice)
Peas
Potatoes (jacket potatoes)
Chickpeas
Pumpkin (butternut squash)
Pumpkin (acorn gourd)
Pumpkin (spaghetti squash)
Carrots
Sweet potatoes
Tomatoes
**Vegetable
s (not recommended)**
Corn

Low GI Fruits (1st Choice) (2 Servings/Day)
Apples
Apricots
Bananas
Blueberries
Blackberries
Strawberries
Guava
Raspberries
Melon (honeydew melon)
Melon (cantaloupe melon)
Melon (watermelon)

Nectarines
Papayas
Peaches
Cranberries
Rhubarb
Grapes
Lemons

Medium GI fruits (2nd choice)
Pears
Figs
Grapefruit
Cherries
Kiwi fruit
Pumpkin
Tangerine
Mango
Oranges
Plums

Meat and Seafood (recommended)
All fish (especially salmon, plaice, herring, tuna, halibut, sole, carp, sardines, mackerel)
All shellfish
Eggs
Chicken (skinless)
Lamb (lean)
Turkey meat (skinless)
Beef (lean and steaks)... rare!
Pork (lean and steaks)... rare!
Sausage (only lean cold cuts)

Dairy Products (Recommended)
Blue cheese
Butter substitute (e.g., ghee)
Buttermilk
Feta cheese
Cream cheese (low in fat)
Greek yogurt
Oat milk
Hazer cheese
Cottage Cheese and Cheddar (Low Fat)
Yogurt (low fat)
Coconut water
Almond milk
Milk (cow's milk, low-fat)
Mozzarella (low fat)
Parmesan cheese
Provolone; Italian sliced cheese (low in fat)
Rice milk
Ricotta cheese (low fat)
Sour cream (low fat)
Sliced cheese (up to 45% fat)
Swiss cheese
Soy milk
Quark (lean)

Dairy Products (not recommended)
Butter
Crème fraîche and sour cream
Fruit curd
Mayonnaise
Milk (full fat)
Rice pudding
Pudding
Cream

Fats / Oils (Approx. 2 tbsp. / Day)
Coconut oil
Flaxseed oil
Olive oil
Rapeseed oil

Nuts, Seeds, etc. (Approx. 20 g / Day)
Cashew nuts
Hazelnuts
Pumpkin seeds
Macadamia
Almonds
Pine nuts
Sesame seeds
Sunflower seeds
Walnuts
Nuts, seeds (not recommended)
Peanuts
All salted nuts

Bread, pasta and other
Cereal products (recommended)
Amaranth
Dark Bread
Barley
Oatmeal
Corn bred
Almond flour
Muesli without sugar
Pasta (whole grain)
Quinoa
Rice (whole grain)
Whole wheat pita
Whole-grain tortillas
Whole grain bread
Wholegrain crispbread
Whole wheat flour
Wheat germ
Cereal products (not recommended)
Croissants
Durum wheat pasta
Potato pancakes
Croquettes
Pancakes
French fries
Rice (peeled)
White bread
Wheat and milk rolls
Zwieback
Snacks (recommended)
Olives

Dried fruits (without sugar)
Dates
Vegetable sticks
Snacks (not recommended)
Sweet and salty baked goods
Sweets
Savory biscuits (chips, flips, etc.)
Sweet dairy products (fruit yogurt, etc.)

Drinks (recommended) - 2-3 l / Day
Fruit juice (freshly squeezed)
Green tea
Herbal tea
Black tea
Water

Drinks (not recommended)
Alcohol
Fruit juices (ready-made juices)
Coffee
Soft drinks

HOW DASH DIET HELPS YOU LOSE WEIGHT AND LOWER BLOOD PRESSURE

Despite not being specifically designed for weight loss, the Dash Diet does indeed help to trim down your weight through various indirect means.
While the DASH diet does not include greater reductions in calories, it influences you to fill up your diet with very nutrient-dense food, instead of calorie-rich food, which easily helps shed a few pounds!
Since you will be on a heavy diet of veggies and fruits, you will be consuming lots of fiber, which is also believed to help in weight loss.
Aside from that, the diet also helps to control your appetite since cleaner, and nutrient-dense foods will keep you satisfied throughout the day! Lower food intake will further contribute to weight loss.
While you are at it, the program will indirectly encourage you to carry out a daily workout to keep your body get healthy and fit. Following the DASH Diet recommendations while working out will significantly enhance the effectiveness of the program.

Understanding the Food Groups
To keep things simple, let me break down the food groups to understand the program's food regime better.
Eat as much as you want:
Grains, such as barley, wheat bread, wheat pasta, etc.
Meats, such as eggs, lean beef, lean chicken, and lean pork.
Seafood, such as fish, shrimp, and salmon.
Fruits such as apples, bananas, cherries, grapes, blackberries, mangoes, etc.
Vegetables, such as artichokes, broccoli, Brussels sprouts, carrots, bell peppers, green beans, etc.

Limit Your Servings:
Healthy vegetable oils, such as canola, corn, olive, etc.
Condiments.
Dairy foods such as Greek yogurt, skim milk, low-fat milk, low-fat cheese.
Nuts, legumes, and seeds such as almonds, cashews, flax seeds, hazelnuts, lentils, pecans, kidney beans.
Red meats.
Eat Rarely:
Sweets, such as beverages, jams, jellies, sugars, sweet yogurt.
Saturated fats such as bacon, coconuts, fatty meats.
Sodium-rich foods such as canned fruits, canned vegetables, gravy pizza, etc.

Understanding Daily Proportions

Controlling your daily portions is crucial when it comes to the Dash Diet program. While the key component here is to keep your sodium intake at a low level, you must consider other things.

Therefore, to maintain properly your DASH diet, you should:

Consume more fruits, low-fat dairy foods, and vegetables.

Eat more whole-grain foods, nuts, poultry, and fish.

Try to limit sodium, sugary drinks, sweets, and red meat, such as beef/pork, etc.

Research has shown that you will get results within just 2 weeks! Alternatively, a different diet, known as DASH-Sodium, calls for cutting down sodium to about 1,500 mg per day (about 2/3 teaspoon).

Generally speaking, the suggested DASH routine includes:

Daily 7-8 servings of grains.

Daily 4-5 servings of vegetables.

Daily 4-5 servings of fruits.

Daily 2-3 servings of low fat/ fat-free dairy products.

Daily 2 or fewer servings of meat/fish/poultry.

4-5 servings per week of nuts, dry beans, and seeds.

Daily 2-3 servings of fats and oil.

And just to give you an idea of what "Each" serving means, here are a few pointers.

The following quantities are to be considered as 1 serving:

½ cup of cooked rice/pasta

1 slice of bread

1 cup of raw fruit or veggies

½ cup of cooked fruit or veggies

8 ounces of milk

3 ounces of cooked meat

1 teaspoon of olive oil/ or any healthy oil

3 ounces of tofu

Salt Alternatives

Letting go of salt might be a little bit difficult for people who are going into this diet for the first time. To make the process a little bit easier, here are some great salt alternatives you should know about! Some of them are used in the recipes in our book, and you may use them if needed.

Sunflower Seeds

Sunflower seeds are excellent salt alternatives, and they give a nice nutty and slightly sweet flavor. You may use the seeds raw or roasted.

Fresh Squeezed Lemon

Lemon is believed to be a nice hybrid between citron and bitter orange. These are packed with Vitamin C, which helps to neutralize damaging free radicals from the system.

Onion Powder

Onion powder is a dehydrated and ground spice made out of an onion bulb for those of you who don't know. The powder is mainly used for seasoning in many spices! Keep in mind that onion powder and onion salt are two different items.

We are using onion powder here. They sport a nice mix of sweet, spice, and a bit of an earthy flavor.

Black Pepper Powder

Black pepper powder is also a salt alternative native to India. You may use it by grinding whole peppercorns!

Cinnamon

Cinnamon is a very well-known and savory spice that comes from the inner bark of trees. Two varieties of cinnamon include Ceylon and Chinese, and they sport a sharp, warm and sweet flavor.

Flavored Vinegar

As we call it in our book, fruit-infused vinegar, or flavored vinegar, is a mixture of vinegar that is combined with fruits to give a nice flavor. These are excellent ingredients to add a bit of flavor to meals without salt. Experimentation might be required to find the perfect fruit blend for you.

As for the process of making the vinegar:

Wash your fruits and slice them well.

Place ½ cup of your fruit in a mason jar.

Top them up with white wine vinegar (or balsamic vinegar).

Let them rest for about 2 weeks.

Strain and use as needed.

The Health Benefits of DASH Diet

Now, before you move forward, let me share some of the incredible health benefits you will enjoy while you are on the program.

Lower Blood Pressure

This is perhaps the main reason why the DASH diet was even invented!

Salt is believed to be very closely related to increasing blood pressure. The purpose of the DASH diet is to closely monitor salt intake, reduce it to very low levels, and improve your overall wellbeing.

Aside from the salt itself, the DASH diet also helps control the levels of potassium, magnesium, and calcium, which altogether plays a great role in lowering blood pressure!

The balanced diet also helps control cholesterol and fat levels in your system, which prevents atherosclerosis, which further helps to keep the arteries healthy and strain-free.

Helps Control Diabetes

Since the Dash Diet helps eliminate empty carbohydrates and starchy food from your diet while avoiding simple sugars, a fine balance between the glucose and insulin level of the body is created that helps prevent diabetes.

Also:

It helps to lower cholesterol levels

Helps in weight loss

It gives you a healthier heart

It helps to prevent osteoporosis

It helps to improve kidney health

It helps to prevent cancer

It helps to prevent depression

The pictures in the book do not represent precisely the recipe meal.

CHAPTER 2.
BREAKFASTS

SHRIMP SKILLET

Preparation Time: 10 minutes
Cooking Time: 25 minutes
Servings: 2

INGREDIENTS

- 2 bell peppers
- 1 red onion
- 1-pound of shrimps, peeled
- ½ teaspoon of white pepper
- ½ teaspoon of paprika
- 1 tablespoon of butter

DIRECTIONS

1. Remove the seeds from the bell peppers and cut the vegetable into wedges.
2. Then place them in the skillet.
3. Add peeled shrimps, white pepper, paprika, and butter.
4. Peel and slice the red onion. Add it in the skillet too.
5. Preheat the oven to 365 ºF.
6. Cover the skillet with foil and secure the edges.
7. Transfer it to the preheated oven and cook for 20 minutes.
8. When the time is over, discard the foil and cook the dish for 5 minutes more. Use ventilation mode if you have.

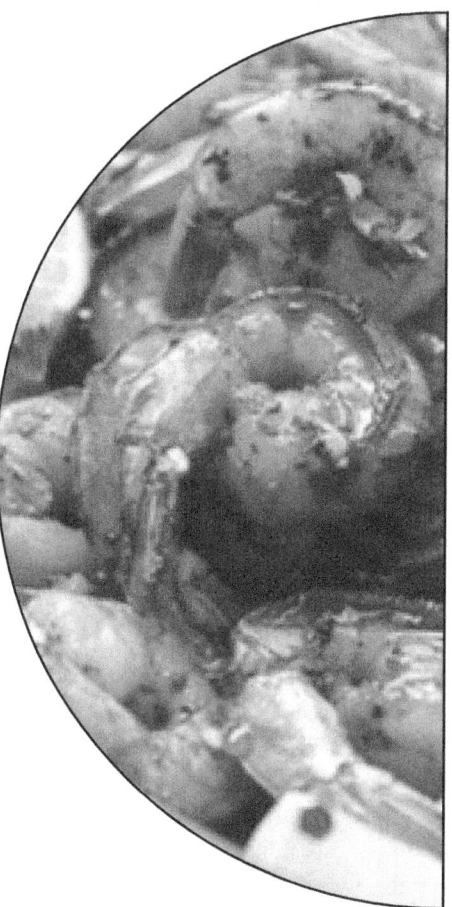

NUTRITION

- Calories: 153
- Fat: 4 g
- Fiber: 1.3 g
- Carbs: 7.3 g
- Protein: 21.5 g

COCONUT YOGURT WITH CHIA SEEDS

Preparation Time: 2 hours
Cooking Time: 10 minutes
Servings: 2

INGREDIENTS

- 1 probiotic capsule, yogurt capsule
- 1 cup of coconut milk
- 1 tablespoon of coconut meat
- 4 tablespoons of chia seeds

DIRECTIONS

1. Pour coconut milk into the saucepan and preheat it until 108 ºF.
2. Then add a probiotic capsule and stir well. Close the lid and leave the coconut milk for 40 minutes.
3. Meanwhile, shred coconut meat.
4. When the time is over, transfer the milk mixture into the cheesecloth and squeeze it. Leave it like this for 40 minutes more or until the liquid from yogurt is squeezed.
5. After this, transfer the yogurt into the serving glasses.
6. Add chia seeds and coconut meat in every glass and mix up well.
7. Let the cooked yogurt rest for 10 minutes before serving.

NUTRITION

- Calories: 177
- Fat: 16.9 g
- Fiber: 3.9 g
- Carbs: 6.5 g
- Protein: 2.6 g

CHIA PUDDING

Preparation Time: 15 minutes
Cooking Time: 3 minutes
Servings: 2

INGREDIENTS

- 2 cups of almond milk
- 8 tablespoons of chia seeds
- 1 oz. of blackberries
- 1 tablespoon of Erythritol

DIRECTIONS

1. Preheat the almond milk for 3 minutes, then remove it from the heat and add chia seeds.
2. Stir gently and add the Erythritol. Mix it up.
3. In the bottom of the serving glasses, put the blackberries.
4. Then pour almond milk mixture over berries. Let the pudding rest for at least 10 minutes before serving.

NUTRITION

- Calories: 331
- Fat: 31.9 g
- Fiber: 6.7 g
- Carbs: 11.8 g
- Protein: 4.6 g

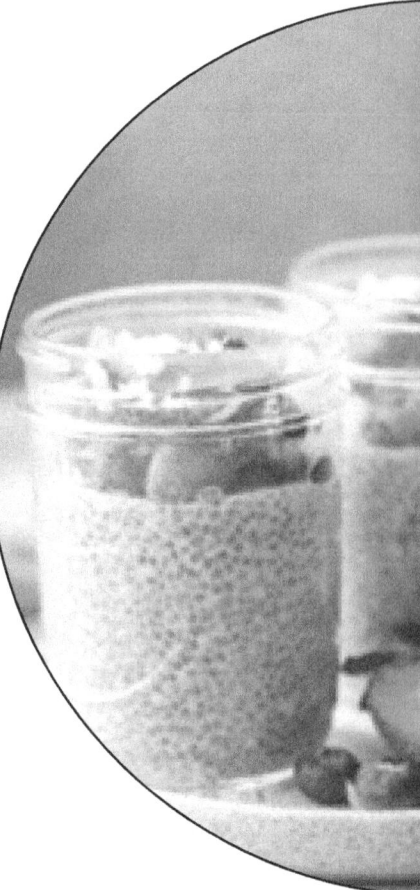

EGG FAT BOMBS

Preparation Time: 10 minutes
Cooking Time: 10 minutes
Servings: 2

INGREDIENTS

- 4 oz. of bacon, sliced
- 4 eggs, boiled
- 1 tablespoon of butter, softened
- ½ teaspoon of salt
- ½ teaspoon of ground black pepper
- 1 tablespoon of mayonnaise

DIRECTIONS

1. Line the tray with the baking paper. Place the bacon on the paper.
2. Preheat the oven to 365 ºF and put the tray inside.
3. Cook the bacon for 10 minutes or until it is light brown.
4. Meanwhile, peel and chop the boiled eggs and transfer them to the mixing bowl.
5. Add the ground black pepper, mayonnaise, and salt.
6. When the bacon is cooked, chill it a little and finely chop.
7. Add the bacon to the egg mixture. Stir it well.
8. Add the softened butter and mix it up again.
9. With the help of the scoop, make medium size balls. Before serving, place them in the fridge for 10 minutes.

NUTRITION

- Calories: 255
- Fat: 20.3 g
- Fiber: 0.1 g
- Carbs: 1.2 g
- Protein: 16.1 g

MORNING "GRITS"

Preparation Time: 10 minutes
Cooking Time: 10 minutes
Servings: 2

INGREDIENTS

- 1 ½ cup of almond milk
- 1 cup of heavy cream, whipped
- 4 tablespoon of chia seeds
- 3 oz. of Parmesan, grated
- ½ teaspoon of chili flakes
- ½ teaspoon of salt
- 1 tablespoon of butter

DIRECTIONS

1. Pour the almond milk into the saucepan and bring it to a boil.
2. Meanwhile, grind the chia seeds with the help of the coffee grinder.
3. Remove the almond milk from the heat and add ground chia seeds.
4. Add whipped cream, chili flakes, and salt. Stir it well and leave for 5 minutes.
5. After this, add butter and grated parmesan. Stir well and preheat it over low heat until the cheese is melted.
6. Stir it again and transfer it to the serving bowls.

NUTRITION

- Calories: 439
- Fat: 42.2 g
- Fiber: 4.4 g
- Carbs: 9.6 g
- Protein: 10.7 g

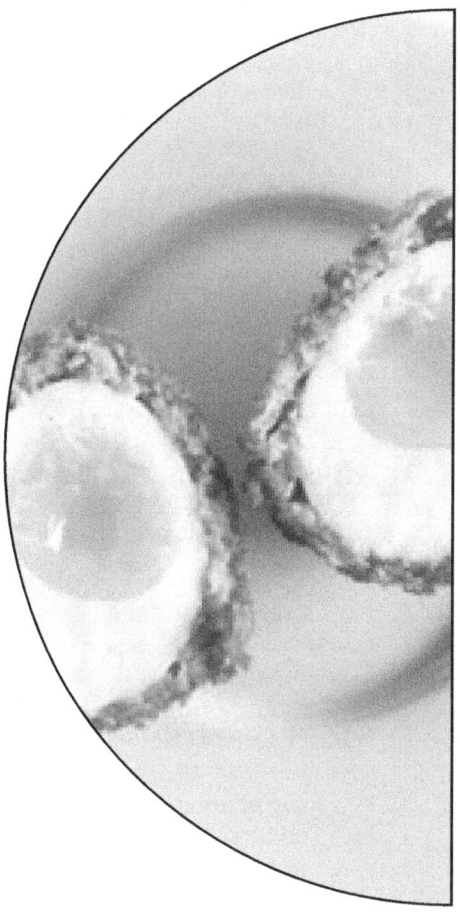

SCOTCH EGGS

Preparation Time: 15 minutes
Cooking Time: 15 minutes
Servings: 2

INGREDIENTS

- 4 eggs, boiled
- 1 ½ cup of ground beef
- 1 tablespoon of onion, grated
- ½ teaspoon of ground black pepper
- ¾ cup of water
- ½ teaspoon of salt
- ½ teaspoon of dried oregano
- ½ teaspoon of dried basil
- 1 tablespoon of butter

DIRECTIONS

1. In the mixing bowl, mix up the ground beef, grated onion, ground black pepper, salt, dried oregano, and basil.
2. Peel the boiled eggs.
3. Make 4 balls from the ground beef mixture.
4. Put peeled eggs inside every ground beef ball and press them gently to get the shape of eggs.
5. Spread the tray with the butter and place ground beef eggs on it.
6. Add water.
7. Preheat oven to 365 ºF and transfer the tray inside.
8. Cook the dish for 15 minutes or until each side of Scotch eggs is light brown.

NUTRITION

- Calories: 188
- Fat: 13.4 g
- Fiber: 0.2 g
- Carbs: 0.9 g
- Protein: 15.4 g

BACON SANDWICH

Preparation Time: 15 minutes
Cooking Time: 20 minutes
Servings: 2

INGREDIENTS

- 1 oz. of bacon, 4 slices
- 4 eggs, separated
- 2 teaspoons of ricotta cheese
- ¾ teaspoon of cream of tartar
- 1 teaspoon of flax meal, ground
- 2 lettuce leaves
- Salt to taste

DIRECTIONS

1. Whisk the egg yolks with 1 teaspoon of ricotta cheese until you get a soft, light, and fluffy mixture.
2. After this, whip together egg whites with remaining ricotta cheese, salt, and cream of tartar. When the mixture is fluffy, add a ground flax meal and stir gently.
3. Preheat the oven to 310 ºF.
4. Gently combine the egg yolks mixture and egg white mixture.
5. Line the tray with baking paper.
6. Make the 4 medium size clouds from the egg mixture using the spoon.
7. Transfer the tray to the oven and cook them for 20 minutes or until they are light brown.
8. Meanwhile, place bacon slices in the skillet and roast them for 1 minute from each side over medium-high heat.
9. Chill the bacon a little.
10. Transfer the cooked and chilled egg clouds to the plate.
11. Place bacon onto 2 clouds and then add lettuce leaves. Cover them with the remaining egg clouds.
12. Secure the sandwiches with toothpicks and transfer them to the serving plate

NUTRITION

- Calories: 218
- Fat: 15.5 g
- Fiber: 0.4 g
- Carbs: 2.3 g
- Protein: 17.2 g

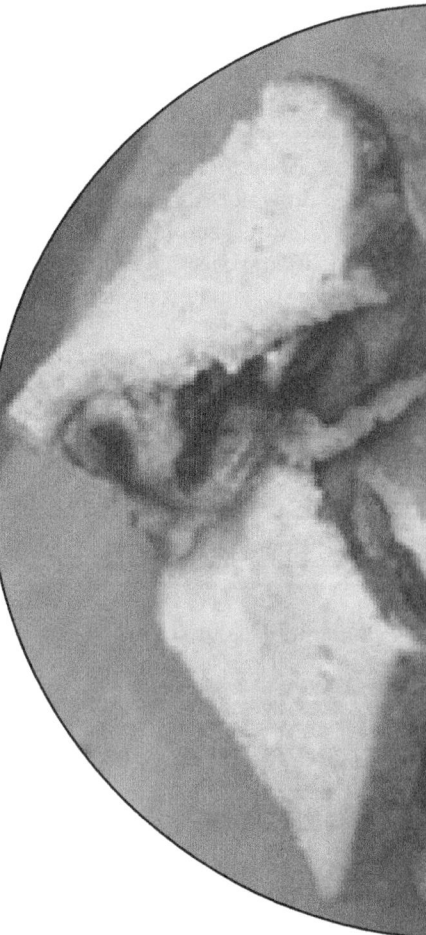

NOATMEAL

Preparation Time: 10 minutes
Cooking Time: 10 minutes
Servings: 2

INGREDIENTS

- 1 cup of organic almond milk
- 2 tablespoons of hemp seeds
- 1 tablespoon of chia seeds, dried
- 1 tablespoon of Erythritol
- 1 tablespoon of almond flakes
- 2 tablespoons of coconut flour
- 1 tablespoon of flax meal
- 1 tablespoon of walnuts, chopped
- ½ teaspoon of vanilla extract
- ¼ teaspoon of ground cinnamon

DIRECTIONS

1. Put all the ingredients except vanilla extract in the saucepan and stir gently.
2. Cook the mixture on low heat for 10 minutes. Stir it constantly.
3. When the mixture starts to be thick, add vanilla extract. Mix it up.
4. Remove the oatmeal from the heat and let it rest a little.

NUTRITION

- Calories: 350
- Fat: 30.4 g
- Fiber: 8.4 g
- Carbs: 16.9 g
- Protein: 9.1 g

BREAKFAST BAKE WITH MEAT

Preparation Time: 10 minutes
Cooking Time: 30 minutes
Servings: 2

INGREDIENTS

- 1 cup of ground beef
- 1 cup of cauliflower, shredded
- ½ cup of coconut cream
- 1 onion, diced
- 1 teaspoon of butter
- ½ teaspoon of salt
- ½ teaspoon of paprika
- ½ teaspoon of garam masala
- 1 tablespoon of fresh cilantro, chopped
- 1 oz. of celery root, grated
- 1 oz. of Cheddar cheese, grated

DIRECTIONS

1. Mix up the garam masala mixture, celery root, paprika, salt, and ground beef.
2. Mix up the shredded cauliflower and salt.
3. Spread the casserole tray with butter.
4. Make the layer of the ground beef mixture inside the casserole tray.
5. Then place the layer of the cauliflower mixture and diced onion.
6. Sprinkle it with grated cheese and fresh cilantro, then, add the coconut cream.
7. Cover the surface of the casserole with the foil and secure the lids.
8. Preheat the oven to 365 ºF.
9. Place the casserole tray in the oven and cook it for 30 minutes.
10. When the time is over, transfer the casserole from the oven, remove the foil and let it chill for 15 minutes.
11. Cut it into the serving and transfer it to the serving bowls.

NUTRITION

- Calories: 192
- Fat: 14.7 g
- Fiber: 2.1 g
- Carbs: 6.5 g
- Protein: 10 g

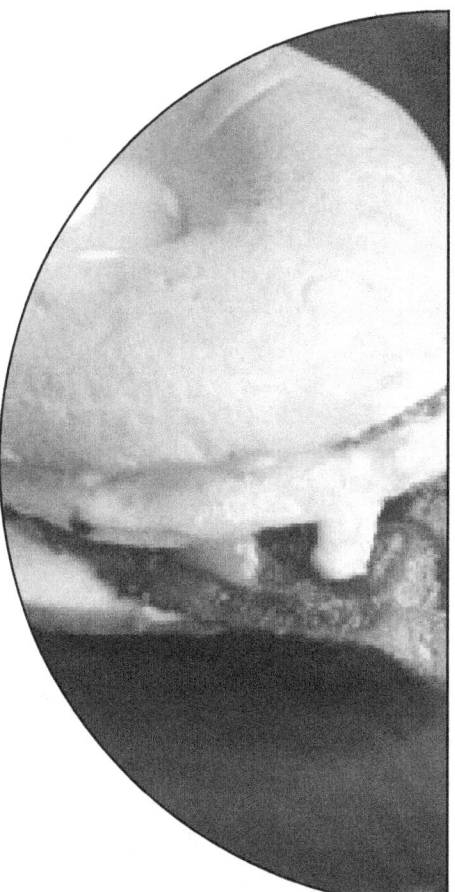

BREAKFAST BAGEL

Preparation Time: 15 minutes
Cooking Time: 30 minutes
Servings: 2

INGREDIENTS

- ½ cup of almond flour
- 1 ½ teaspoon of xanthan gum
- 1 egg, beaten
- 3 oz. of Parmesan, grated
- ½ teaspoon of cumin seeds
- 1 teaspoon of cream cheese
- 1 teaspoon of butter, melted

DIRECTIONS

1. In the mixing bowl, mix up the almond flour, xanthan gum, and egg.
2. Stir it until homogenous.
3. Put the cheese in a separate bowl and add the cream cheese.
4. Microwave the mixture until it is melted. Stir it well.
5. Combine the cheese mixture and almond flour mixture and knead the dough.
6. Roll the dough into the log.
7. Cut the log into 3 pieces and make bagels.
8. Line the tray with baking paper and place bagels on it.
9. Brush the bagels with melted butter and sprinkle with cumin seeds.
10. Preheat the oven to 365 ºF.
11. Put the tray with bagels in the oven and cook for 30 minutes.
12. Check if the bagels are cooked with the help of the toothpicks.
13. Cut the bagels and spread them with your favorite spread.

NUTRITION

- Calories: 262
- Fat: 18.6 g
- Fiber: 8.7 g
- Carbs: 12 g
- Protein: 15.1 g

EGG AND VEGETABLE HASH

Preparation Time: 8 minutes
Cooking Time: 20 minutes
Servings: 2

INGREDIENTS

- 4 eggs
- 1 white onion, diced
- 6 oz. of turnip, chopped
- 2 bell peppers, chopped
- 1 garlic clove, peeled, diced
- 1 jalapeno pepper, sliced
- 5 oz. of Swiss cheese, grated
- 1 tablespoon of lemon juice
- 1 tablespoon of canola oil
- ½ teaspoon of Taco seasoning

DIRECTIONS

1. Beat the eggs in the bowl and whisk gently.
2. Then pour canola oil into the pan and preheat it.
3. Add chopped turnips and white onion. Mix up the vegetables and cook them for 5 minutes over medium heat. Stir them from time to time.
4. Then add diced garlic and chopped peppers.
5. Sprinkle the vegetables with taco seasoning and mix up well.
6. Add lemon juice and close the lid. Cook it for 5 minutes more.
7. Then pour the whisked egg mixture over the vegetables. Sprinkle with the grated cheese.
8. Close the lid and cook it on low heat for 10 minutes.
9. It is recommended to serve the dish hot.

NUTRITION

- Calories: 184
- Fat: 12 g
- Fiber: 1.5 g
- Carbs: 8.7 g
- Protein: 11 g

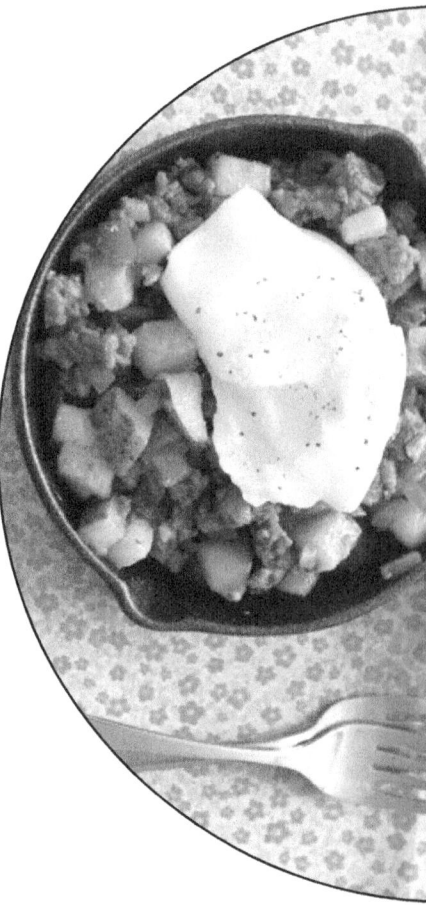

COWBOY SKILLET

Preparation Time: 5 minutes
Cooking Time: 15 minutes
Servings: 2

INGREDIENTS

- 1 cup of rutabaga, chopped
- 3 eggs, whisked
- ½ cup of fresh cilantro, chopped
- 6 oz. of chorizo, chopped
- 1 tablespoon of olive oil
- ¾ cup of heavy cream

DIRECTIONS

1. Put the rutabaga in the skillet. Add the olive oil and chorizo.
2. Mix the mixture up and close the lid. Cook it for 5 minutes over medium heat.
3. When the rutabaga becomes tender add the whisked eggs and chopped cilantro.
4. Add heavy cream and stir the meal with the help of a spatula.
5. Close the lid and sauté it for 10 minutes over medium-low heat.

NUTRITION

- Calories: 362
- Fat: 31.5 g
- Fiber: 1 g
- Carbs: 4.7 g
- Protein: 15.4 g

FETA QUICHE

Preparation Time: 15 minutes
Cooking Time: 25 minutes
Servings: 2

INGREDIENTS

- 8 oz. of Feta cheese, crumbled
- 5 eggs, whisked
- 1 cup of spinach, chopped
- 1 garlic clove, diced
- 1 white onion, diced
- 1 teaspoon of butter
- 5 oz. of Mozzarella, chopped
- ½ teaspoon of chili flakes
- 1 teaspoon of paprika
- ½ teaspoon of white pepper
- ½ cup of whipped cream

DIRECTIONS

1. Toss the butter in the skillet and preheat it.
2. Add the diced garlic and onion and cook it over medium heat until the vegetables are soft.
3. Transfer the cooked vegetables to the mixing bowl. Add the crumbled cheese, whisked eggs, spinach, chopped Mozzarella, chili flakes, paprika, white pepper, and the whipped cream.
4. Mix the mixture well and transfer it in the non-sticky mold. Flatten it gently with the spatula.
5. Place the mold in the preheated to 365 ºF oven and cook quiche for 25 minutes.
6. Chill the quiche a little and then cut into the servings.

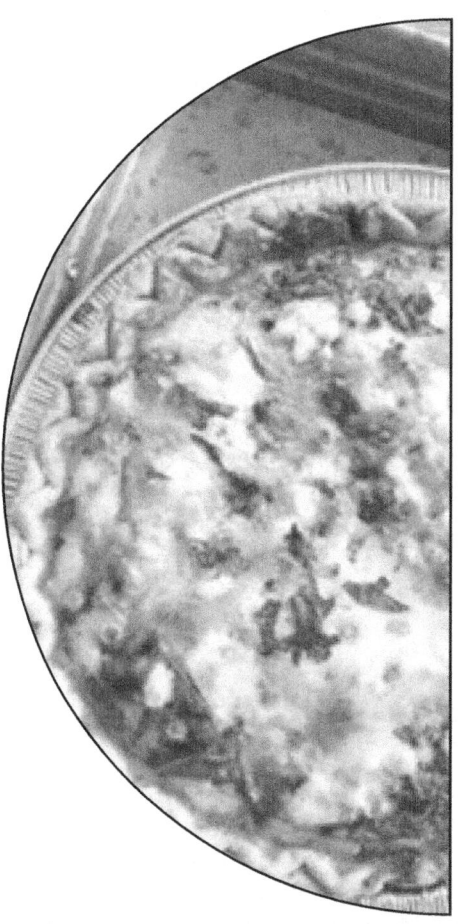

BACON PANCAKES

Preparation Time: 10 minutes
Cooking Time: 10 minutes
Servings: 2

INGREDIENTS

- 3 oz. of bacon, chopped
- ½ cup of almond flour
- ¾ cup of heavy cream
- ½ teaspoon of baking powder
- ¼ teaspoon of salt
- 1 egg, whisked

DIRECTIONS

1. Place the chopped bacon in the skillet and cook it for 5-6 minutes over medium-high heat. The cooked bacon should be a little bit crunchy.
2. Meanwhile, mix up the almond flour, heavy cream, salt, baking powder, and whisked egg. When the mixture is smooth, the batter is cooked.
3. Add the cooked bacon to the batter and stir it gently with the help of the spoon.
4. Don't clean the skillet after the bacon. Ladle the bacon batter in the skillet and make the pancake.
5. Cook it for 1 minute from one side and then flip onto another side.
6. Cook it for 1.5 minutes more.
7. Make the same steps with the remaining batter.
8. Transfer the pancakes to the serving plate.

WAFFLES

Preparation Time: 10 minutes
Cooking Time: 10 minutes
Servings: 2

INGREDIENTS

- 2 tablespoons of butter, melted
- 4 eggs, whisked
- 1 teaspoon of baking powder
- 1 teaspoon of lemon juice
- 1 cup of almond flour
- ½ teaspoon of vanilla extract
- 1 tablespoon of Erythritol
- ¾ cup of organic almond milk

DIRECTIONS

1. In the mixing bowl, combine all the ingredients.
2. Whisk the smooth and homogenous batter.
3. Preheat the waffle maker well.
4. Pour enough of the batter into the waffle maker. Flatten it gently to get a waffle. Close it and cook until lightly golden.
5. Repeat the same steps with all remaining batter.
6. Serve the waffles warm.

NUTRITION

- Calories: 167
- Fat: 13.7 g
- Fiber: 1 g
- Carbs: 3 g
- Protein: 7.4 g

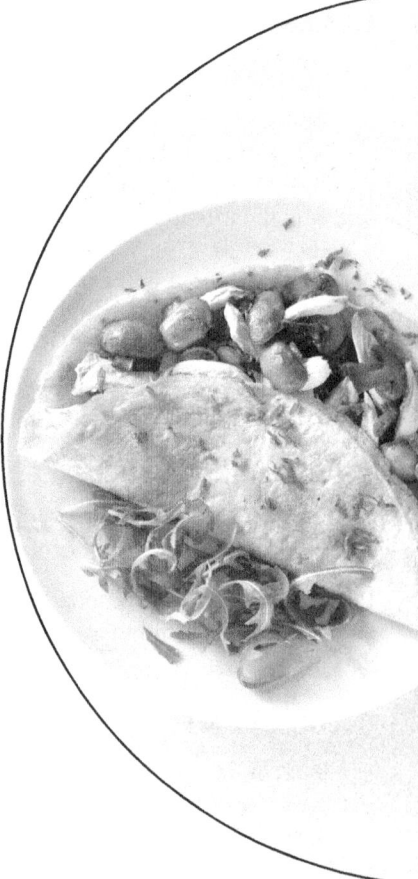

ROLLED OMELETTE WITH MUSHROOMS

Preparation Time: 10 minutes
Cooking Time: 20 minutes
Servings: 2

INGREDIENTS

- 1 cup of mushrooms, chopped
- ½ white onion, sliced
- ½ teaspoon of tomato paste
- 2 tablespoons of water
- ½ teaspoon of salt
- ½ teaspoon of cayenne pepper
- ¾ teaspoon of chili flakes
- 3 eggs, beaten
- 1 tablespoon of cream cheese
- 1 teaspoon of butter
- 1 teaspoon of avocado oil

DIRECTIONS

1. Pour the avocado oil into the skillet and preheat it.
2. Add the chopped mushrooms and sliced onion.
3. Then add the tomato paste and water. Stir the ingredients and sauté them with the closed lid for 10 minutes.
4. Transfer the cooked vegetables to the mixing bowl.
5. Whisk the cream cheese, eggs, chili flakes, cayenne pepper, and salt.
6. Toss the butter in the skillet and melt it.
7. Add the egg mixture. Close the lid.
8. Cook it for 10 minutes over medium-low heat.
9. Then spread the mushroom mixture over the cooked omelet and roll it.
10. Cut the cooked meal into 3 parts and transfer it on the serving plates.

NUTRITION

- Calories: 102
- Fat: 7.1 g
- Fiber: 0.8 g
- Carbs: 3.4 g
- Protein: 6.8 g

QUICHE LORRAINE QUICHE LORRAINE

Preparation Time: 15 minutes
Cooking Time: 18 minutes
Servings: 2

INGREDIENTS

- 1/3 cup of butter, softened
- 1 cup of almond flour
- ½ teaspoon of salt
- 1 oz. of bacon, chopped
- 1 white onion, diced
- 1/3 cup of heavy cream
- 5 oz. of Swiss cheese, grated
- 2 eggs, whisked
- ½ teaspoon of ground black pepper
- 1 teaspoon of olive oil

DIRECTIONS

1. Make the quiche crust: combine the softened butter, almond flour, and salt. Knead the dough. Roll it up.
2. Place it in the pie pan and flatten to get the piecrust. Pin it with the help of the fork.
3. Preheat the oven to 360 °F and put the pan with the piecrust inside. Cook it for 18 minutes.
4. Meanwhile, pour olive oil into the skillet.
5. Add diced onion and chopped bacon. Cook the ingredients for 5-6 minutes or until they are soft.
6. When the piecrust is cooked, remove it from the oven and chill a little.
7. Spread it with the onion mixture and sprinkle it with Swiss cheese.
8. Then combine the whisked eggs and heavy cream.
9. Pour the liquid over the cheese.
10. Transfer the pie to the oven and cook for 10 minutes at 355 °F.
11. Chill the cooked quiche well and cut into the servings.

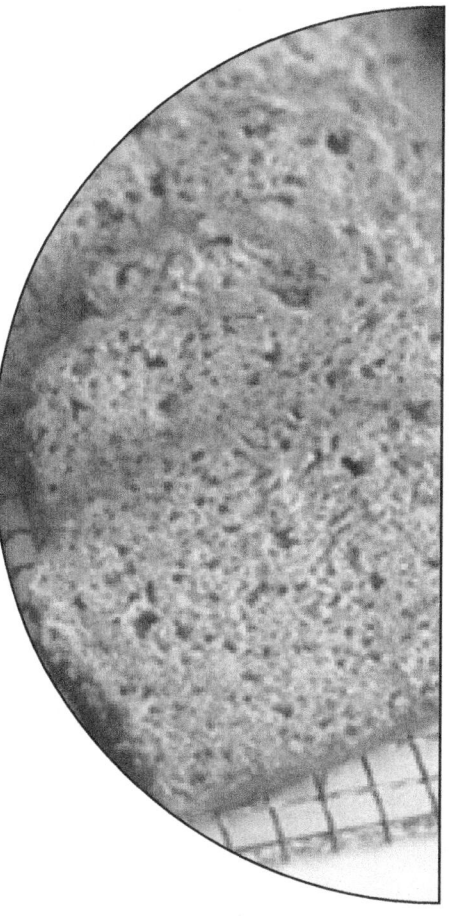

BREAKFAST ZUCCHINI BREAD

Preparation Time: 15 minutes
Cooking Time: 50 minutes
Servings: 2

INGREDIENTS

- ½ cup of walnuts, chopped
- 1 teaspoon of baking powder
- 1 tablespoon of lemon juice
- 1 tablespoon of flax meal
- 1 ½ cup of almond flour
- 1 teaspoon of xanthan gum
- 1 tablespoon of butter, melted
- 3 eggs, beaten
- 1 teaspoon of salt

DIRECTIONS

1. Preheat oven to 360 °F.
2. In the mixing bowl, combine all wet ingredients. Whisk the mixture well.
3. Then add baking powder, flax meal, almond flour, zucchini, xanthan gum, and salt.
4. Mix up the mixture. Add chopped walnuts and stir it well. You will get a liquid, but thick dough. Check if you add all the ingredients.
5. Transfer the dough into the non-sticky loaf mold and flatten its surface with the spatula.
6. Place the bread in the oven and cook for 50 minutes.
7. Check if the bread is cooked with the help of the toothpick—if it is clean—the bread is cooked.
8. Remove the zucchini bread from the oven and chill well, then remove it from the mold and let it chill totally.

GRANOLA

Preparation Time: 10 minutes
Cooking Time: 25 minutes
Servings: 2

INGREDIENTS

- 4 tablespoons of walnuts
- 3 tablespoons of pecans
- 3 tablespoons of hazelnuts
- 1 tablespoon of chia seeds
- 2 tablespoons of pumpkin seeds
- 2 tablespoons of flax meal
- 1 tablespoon of coconut shred
- 1 tablespoon of Erythritol
- 2 tablespoons of almond butter
- 1 tablespoon of peanut butter

DIRECTIONS

1. Chop the walnuts, pecans, hazelnuts, pumpkin seeds, and transfer to the mixing bowl.
2. Add the chia seeds, flax meal, coconut shred, Erythritol, almond butter, and peanut butter. Blend the mixture. The mass should be sticky.
3. Preheat the oven to 300 ºF.
4. Line the tray with parchment.
5. Transfer the nut mixture into the parchment and flatten it into the layer.
6. Place the tray in the oven and cook it for 25 minutes.
7. When the time is over, remove the tray from the oven and chill granola.
8. Cut it into medium size pieces. Store granola in the glass jar with the closed lid.

NUTRITION

- Calories: 373
- Fat: 34.5 g
- Fiber: 7.4 g
- Carbs: 11.7 g
- Protein: 11.6 g

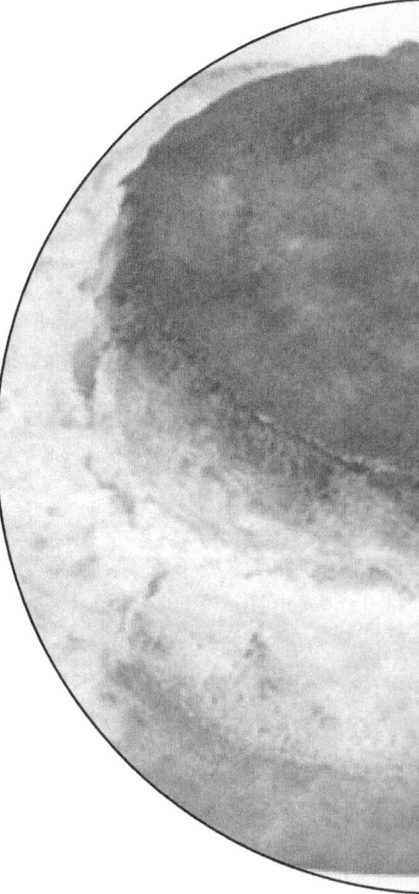

CHEDDAR SOUFFLÉ

Preparation Time: 10 minutes
Cooking Time: 25 minutes
Servings: 2

INGREDIENTS

- 2 oz. of Cheddar cheese, grated
- ½ teaspoon of ground black pepper
- ½ teaspoon of salt
- ½ cup of almond milk
- ½ onion
- 1 bay leaf
- ¼ teaspoon of peppercorn
- 1 tablespoon of coconut shred
- 2 teaspoon of butter, melted
- 2 eggs
- 1 teaspoon of coconut oil
- 2 cups of almond flour
- ½ teaspoon of paprika

DIRECTIONS

1. Brush the ramekins with coconut oil and sprinkle with coconut shred.
2. Then pour ¼ cup of the almond milk into the saucepan. Add onion and peppercorns.
3. Bring it to a boil.
4. Remove the onion and peppercorns.
5. Toss the butter in the pan and add the almond flour. Stir it well until smooth.
6. Add the salt, ground black pepper, and paprika. Mix up well.
7. After this, separate egg yolk and egg whites.
8. Add the egg yolks to the almond flour mixture. Stir it well.
9. Add the other ¼ cup of almond milk and start to preheat it. Stir it all the time until the mixture is smooth.
10. After this, whisk the egg whites until the strong peaks.
11. Add the grated Cheddar to the almond flour mixture. Mix it up.
12. Then chill the mixture a little.
13. Add the egg whites and mix up gently.
14. Preheat the oven to 365 ºF.
15. Place the cheese mixture into the prepared ramekins and transfer it on the tray.
16. Put the tray in the preheated oven and cook for 15 minutes.
17. When the soufflé is cooked, it will have a light brown color.

NUTRITION

- Calories: 384
- Fat: 34.3 g
- Fiber: 2.4 g
- Carbs: 7.6 g
- Protein: 14.5 g

MEDITERRANEAN OMELETTE

Preparation Time: 5 minutes
Cooking Time: 10 minutes
Servings: 2

INGREDIENTS

- 3 eggs, beaten
- 1 tablespoon of ricotta cheese
- 2 oz. of feta cheese, chopped
- 1 tomato, chopped
- 1 teaspoon of butter
- ½ teaspoon of salt
- 1 tablespoon of scallions, chopped

DIRECTIONS

1. Mix up the ricotta cheese and eggs. Add salt and scallions.
2. Toss the butter in the skillet and melt it.
3. Pour ½ part of the whisked egg mixture in the skillet and cook it for 5-6 minutes or until it is solid—the omelet is cooked.
4. Then transfer the omelet to the plate.
5. Make the second omelet with the remaining egg mixture.
6. Sprinkle each omelet with Feta and tomatoes. Roll them.

NUTRITION

- Calories: 203
- Fat: 15.2 g
- Fiber: 0.5 g
- Carbs: 3.5 g
- Protein: 13.6 g

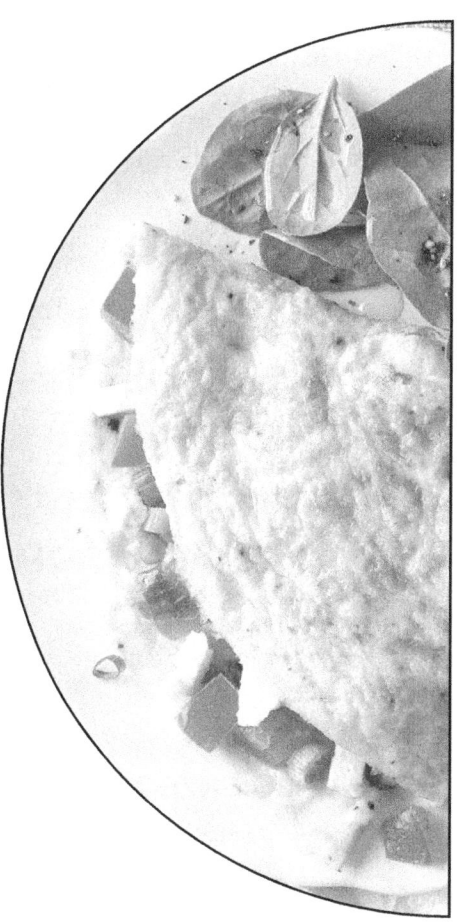

CHICKEN FRITTERS

Preparation Time: 10 minutes
Cooking Time: 8 minutes
Servings: 2

INGREDIENTS

- 1-pound of chicken fillet, finely chopped
- 2 tablespoons of almond flour
- 1 egg, beaten
- 1 teaspoon of dried dill
- 1 teaspoon of dried oregano
- ½ teaspoon of salt
- 1 teaspoon of minced garlic
- 1 tablespoon of olive oil

DIRECTIONS

1. Put the finely chopped chicken fillet and almond flour in the mixing bowl.
2. Add beaten egg, dried dill, oregano, salt, and minced garlic. Mix it up.
3. Make the fritters.
4. Pour olive oil into the skillet and preheat it until hot.
5. Add the fritters and cook them for 4 minutes from each side over medium heat.
6. Dry the fritters with the help of the paper towel and transfer them to the serving bowl.

NUTRITION

- Calories: 284
- Fat: 14.8 g
- Fiber: 0.6 g
- Carbs: 1.4 g
- Protein: 35.1 g

EGGS IN PORTOBELLO MUSHROOM HATS

Preparation Time: 10 minutes
Cooking Time: 15 minutes
Servings: 2

INGREDIENTS

- 4 Portobello caps
- 4 quail eggs
- ½ teaspoon of dried parsley
- ¾ teaspoon of salt
- 1 teaspoon of butter, melted

DIRECTIONS

1. Brush Portobello caps with melted butter from all sides.
2. Line the tray with baking paper.
3. Put Portobello caps on the tray.
4. Beat the quail eggs into the mushroom caps and sprinkle them with salt and dried parsley.
5. Transfer the tray in the preheated to the 355 ºF oven. Cook the mushrooms for 15 minutes.
6. Chill the meal a little and transfer on the serving plates.

NUTRITION

- Calories: 46
- Fat: 3.9 g
- Fiber: 0 g
- Carbs: 0.2 g
- Protein: 2.4 g

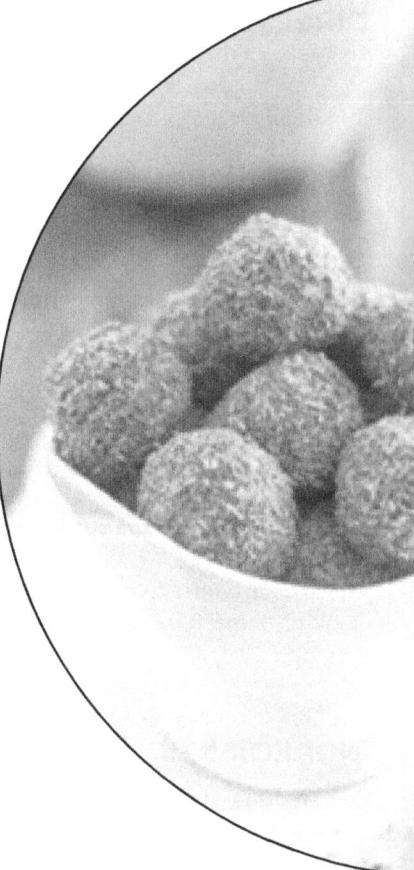

MATCHA FAT BOMBS

Preparation Time: 15 minutes
Cooking Time: 5 minutes
Servings: 2

INGREDIENTS

- ½ cup of cashew butter
- 1 cup of coconut butter
- ¼ cup of coconut cream
- 2 tablespoons of matcha green tea
- ¼ teaspoon of ground cinnamon
- ½ cup of coconut shred

DIRECTIONS

1. Put the cashew butter, coconut butter, coconut cream, ½ tablespoon of matcha green tea, and ground cinnamon in the mixing bowl.
2. Blend the mixture with the hand blender until you get a homogenous and fluffy mass.
3. In the separated bowl, combine the coconut shred and remaining matcha green tea.
4. Make the balls from the coconut butter mixture with the help of the scooper.
5. Then coat every ball in the coconut shred green mixture.
6. Transfer the meal on the plates and store them in the cold place -fridge.

NUTRITION

- Calories: 222
- Fat: 20.7 g
- Fiber: 4.1 g
- Carbs: 9.2 g
- Protein: 3.6 g

SALMON OMELET

Preparation Time: 15 minutes
Cooking Time: 5 minutes
Servings: 2

INGREDIENTS

- 3 eggs
- 1 smoked salmon
- 3 links of pork sausage
- ¼ cup of onions
- ¼ cup of provolone cheese

DIRECTIONS

1. Whisk the eggs and pour them into a skillet.
2. Follow the standard method for making an omelette.
3. Add the onions, salmon and cheese before turning the omelet over.
4. Sprinkle the omelet with cheese and serve with the sausages on the side.
5. Serve!

NUTRITION

- Calories: 346
- Fat: 11.5 g
- Fiber: 3.4 g
- Carbs: 11.5 g
- Protein: 5.6 g

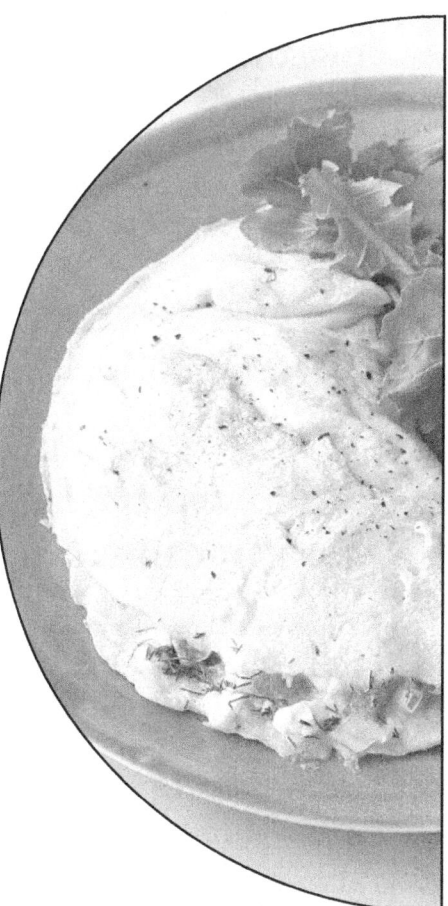

BLACK'S BANGIN' CASSEROLE

Preparation Time: 40 minutes
Cooking Time: 25-35 minutes
Servings: 2

INGREDIENTS

- 5 eggs
- 3 tablespoons of chunky tomato sauce
- 2 tablespoons of heavy cream
- 2 tablespoons of grated parmesan cheese

DIRECTIONS

1. Preheat your oven to 350 °F/175 °C.
2. Combine the eggs and cream in a bowl.
3. Mix in the tomato sauce and add the cheese.
4. Spread into a glass-baking dish and bake for 25-35 minutes.
5. Top with extra cheese.
6. Enjoy!

NUTRITION

- Calories: 346
- Fat: 11.5 g
- Fiber: 3.4 g
- Carbs: 11.5 g
- Protein: 5.6 g

HASH BROWN

Preparation Time: 20 minutes
Cooking Time: 5 minutes
Servings: 2

INGREDIENTS

- 12 oz. of grated fresh cauliflower -about ½ a medium-sized head
- 4 slices of bacon, chopped
- 3 oz. of onion, chopped
- 1 tablespoon of butter, softened

DIRECTIONS

1. In a skillet, sauté the bacon and onion until brown.
2. Add in the cauliflower and stir until tender and browned.
3. Add the butter steadily as it cooks.
4. Season to taste with salt and pepper.
5. Enjoy!

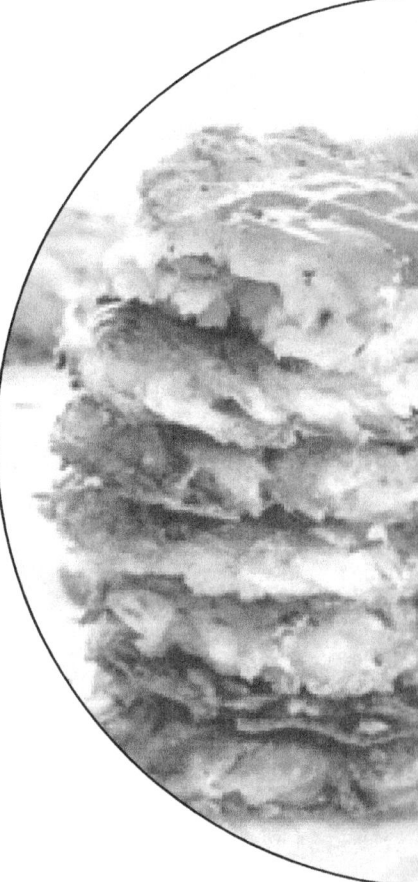

BACON CUPS

Preparation Time: 40 minutes
Cooking Time: 20 minutes
Servings: 2

INGREDIENTS

- 2 eggs
- 1 slice of tomato
- 3 slices of bacon
- 2 slices of ham
- 2 teaspoon of grated parmesan cheese

DIRECTIONS

1. Preheat your oven to 375 °F/190°C.
2. Cook the bacon for half of the directed time.
3. Slice the bacon strips in half and line 2 greased muffin tins with 3 half-strips of bacon
4. Put one slice of ham and a half portion of tomato in each muffin tin on top of the bacon
5. Crack one egg on top of the tomato in each muffin tin and sprinkle each with half a teaspoon of grated parmesan cheese.
6. Bake for 20 minutes.
7. Remove and let cool.
8. Serve!

SPINACH EGGS AND CHEESE

Preparation Time: 40 minutes
Cooking Time: 25-30 minutes
Servings: 2

INGREDIENTS
- 3 whole eggs
- 3 oz. of cottage cheese
- 3-4 oz. of chopped spinach
- ¼ cup of parmesan cheese
- ¼ cup of milk

DIRECTIONS
1. Preheat your oven to 375 °F/190 °C.
2. In a large bowl, whisk the eggs, cottage cheese, parmesan and milk.
3. Mix in the spinach.
4. Transfer to a small, greased oven dish.
5. Sprinkle the cheese on top.
6. Bake for 25-30 minutes.
7. Let it cool for 5 minutes and serve.

NUTRITION
- Calories: 346
- Fat: 11.5 g
- Fiber: 3.4 g
- Carbs: 11.5 g
- Protein: 5.6 g

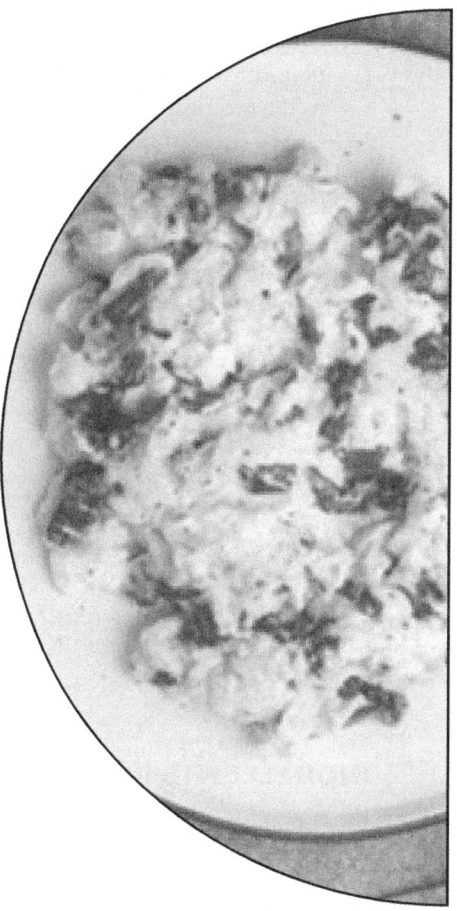

FRIED EGGS

Preparation Time: 7 minutes
Cooking Time: 5 minutes
Servings: 2

INGREDIENTS
- 2 eggs
- 3 slices of bacon

DIRECTIONS
1. Heat some oil in a deep fryer at 375 °F/190°C.
2. Fry the bacon.
3. In a small bowl, add the 2 eggs.
4. Quickly add the eggs into the center of the fryer.
5. Using two spatulas form the egg into a ball while frying.
6. Fry for 2-3 minutes until it stops bubbling.
7. Place on a paper towel and allow draining.
8. Enjoy!

NUTRITION
- Calories: 216
- Fat: 11.5 g
- Fiber: 3.4 g
- Carbs: 11.5 g
- Protein: 5.6 g

TOASTIES

Preparation Time: 30 minutes
Cooking Time: 15-20 minutes
Servings: 2

INGREDIENTS

- ¼ cup of milk or cream
- 2 sausages, boiled
- 3 eggs
- 1 slice of bread, sliced lengthwise
- 4 tablespoons of cheese, grated
- Sea salt to taste
- Chopped fresh herbs and steamed broccoli [optional]

DIRECTIONS

1. Preheat your Air Fryer at 360 °F and set the timer for 5 minutes.
2. In the meantime, scramble the eggs in a bowl and add in the milk.
3. Grease three muffin cups with a cooking spray. Divide the egg mixture into three and pour equal amounts into each cup.
4. Slice the sausages and drop them, along with the slices of bread, into the egg mixture. Add the cheese on top and a little salt as desired.
5. Transfer the cups to the fryer and cook for 15-20 minutes, depending on how firm you would like them. When ready, remove them from the fryer, serve with fresh herbs and steam broccoli if you prefer.
6.

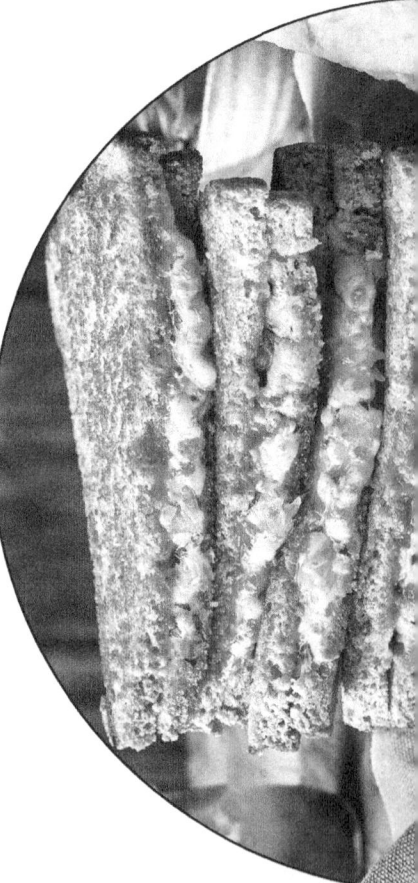

EGG BAKED OMELET

Preparation Time: 15 minutes
Cooking Time: 10 minutes
Servings: 2

INGREDIENTS

- 1 tablespoon of ricotta cheese
- 1 tablespoon of chopped parsley
- 1 tsp. olive oil
- 3 eggs
- ¼ cup chopped spinach
- ¼ cup ricotta cheese
- Salt and pepper to taste

DIRECTIONS

1. Set your Air Fryer at 330 °F and allow it to warm with the olive oil inside.
2. In a bowl, beat the eggs with a fork and sprinkle some salt and pepper as desired.
3. Add in the ricotta, spinach, and parsley and then transfer to the Air Fryer. Cook for 10 minutes before serving.

BREAKFAST OMELET

Preparation Time: 30 minutes
Cooking Time: 15 minutes
Servings: 2

INGREDIENTS

- 1 large onion, chopped
- 2 tablespoons of cheddar cheese, grated
- 3 eggs
- ½ teaspoon of soy sauce
- Salt
- Pepper powder
- Cooking spray

DIRECTIONS

1. In a bowl, mix the salt, pepper powder, soy sauce and eggs with a whisk.
2. Take a small pan small enough to fit inside the Air Fryer and spritz with cooking spray. Spread the chopped onion across the bottom of the pan, and then transfer the pan to the Fryer. Cook at 355°F for 6-7 minutes, ensuring the onions turn translucent.
3. Add the egg mixture on top of the onions, coating everything well. Add the cheese on top, and then resume cooking for another 5 or 6 minutes.
4. Take care when taking the pan out of the fryer. Enjoy with some toasted bread.

NUTRITION

- Calories: 346
- Fat: 11.5 g
- Fiber: 3.4 g
- Carbs: 11.5 g
- Protein: 5.6 g

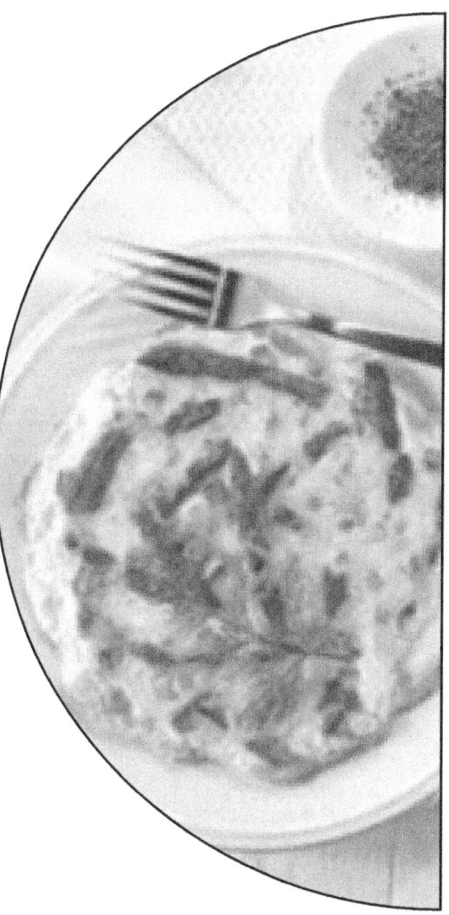

COFFEE DONUTS

Preparation Time: 20 minutes
Cooking Time: 10 minutes
Servings: 2

INGREDIENTS

- 1 cup of almond flour
- ¼ cup of stevia
- ½ teaspoon of salt
- 1 teaspoon of baking powder
- 1 tablespoon of aquafaba
- 1 tablespoon of sunflower oil
- ¼ cup of coffee

DIRECTIONS

1. In a large bowl, combine the stevia, salt, flour, and baking powder.
2. Add in the coffee, aquafaba, and sunflower oil and mix until a dough is formed. Leave the dough to rest in and the refrigerator.
3. Set your Air Fryer at 400 °F to heat up.
4. Remove the dough from the fridge and divide up, kneading each section into a doughnut.
5. Put the doughnuts inside the air fryer, ensuring not to overlap any. Fry for 6 minutes. Do not shake the basket to make sure the doughnuts hold their shape.

NUTRITION

- Calories: 346
- Fat: 11.5 g
- Fiber: 3.4 g
- Carbs: 11.5 g
- Protein: 5.6 g

TACO WRAPS

Preparation Time: 30 minutes
Cooking Time: 15 minutes
Servings: 2

INGREDIENTS

- 1 tablespoon of water
- 4 pieces of commercial vegan nuggets, chopped
- 1 small yellow onion, diced
- 1 small red bell pepper, chopped
- 2 cobs of grilled corn kernels
- 4 large corn tortillas
- Mixed greens for garnish

DIRECTIONS

1. Preheat your Air Fryer at 400 °F.
2. Over medium heat, water-sauté the nuggets with the onions, corn kernels and bell peppers in a skillet, then remove from the heat.
3. Fill the tortillas with the nuggets and vegetables and fold them up. Transfer to the inside of the fryer and cook for 15 minutes. Once crispy, serve immediately, garnished with the mixed greens.

NUTRITION

- Calories: 287
- Fat: 11.5 g
- Fiber: 3.4 g
- Carbs: 11.5 g
- Protein: 5.6 g

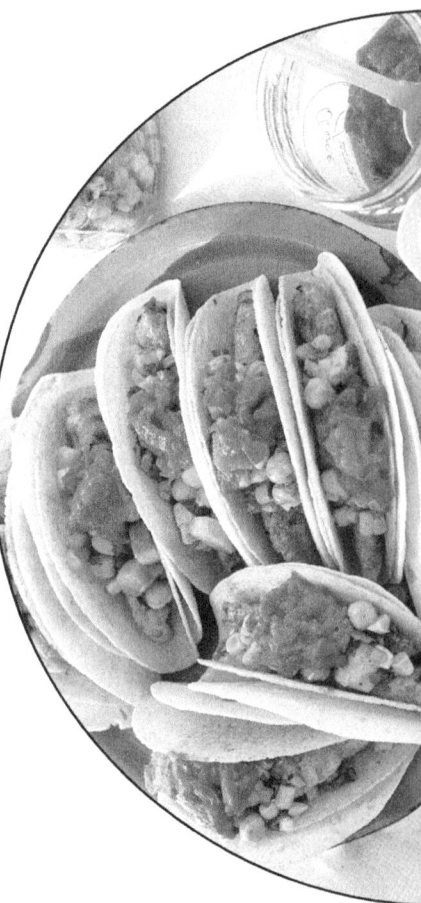

BISTRO WEDGES

Preparation Time: 20 minutes
Cooking Time: 15 minutes
Servings: 2

INGREDIENTS

- 1 lb. of fingerling potatoes, cut into wedges
- 1 teaspoon of extra virgin olive oil
- ½ teaspoon of garlic powder
- Salt and pepper to taste
- ½ cup of raw cashews, soaked in water overnight
- ½ teaspoon of ground turmeric
- ½ teaspoon of paprika
- 1 tablespoon of nutritional yeast
- 1 teaspoon of fresh lemon juice
- 2 tablespoons of to ¼ cup water
- ¼ cup of parmesan cheese

DIRECTIONS

1. Preheat your Air Fryer at 400 °F.
2. In a bowl, toss the potato wedges, olive oil, garlic powder, and salt and pepper, making sure to coat the potatoes well.
3. Transfer the potatoes to the basket of your fryer and fry for 10 minutes.
4. In the meantime, prepare the cheese sauce. Pulse the cashews, turmeric, paprika, nutritional yeast, lemon juice, and water together in a food processor. Add more water to achieve your desired consistency.
5. When the potatoes are finished cooking, move them to a small bowl to fit inside the fryer and add the cheese sauce on top. Cook for an additional 3 minutes.

NUTRITION

- Calories: 346
- Fat: 11.5 g
- Fiber: 3.4 g
- Carbs: 11.5 g
- Protein: 5.6 g

SPINACH BALLS

Preparation Time: 20 minutes
Cooking Time: 10 minutes
Servings: 2

INGREDIENTS

- 1 carrot, peeled and grated
- 1 package fresh spinach, blanched and chopped
- ½ onion, chopped
- 1 egg, beaten
- ½ teaspoon of garlic powder
- 1 teaspoon of garlic, minced
- 1 teaspoon of salt
- ½ teaspoon of black pepper
- 1 tablespoon of nutritional yeast
- 1 tablespoon of almond flour
- 2 slices of bread, toasted

DIRECTIONS

1. In a food processor, pulse the toasted bread to form breadcrumbs. Transfer into a shallow dish or bowl.
2. In a bowl, mix all the other ingredients.
3. Use your hands to shape the mixture into small-sized balls. Roll the balls in the breadcrumbs, ensuring to cover them well.
4. Put in the Air Fryer and cook at 390°F for 10 minutes.

NUTRITION

- Calories: 278
- Fat: 11.5 g
- Fiber: 3.4 g
- Carbs: 11.5 g
- Protein: 5.6 g

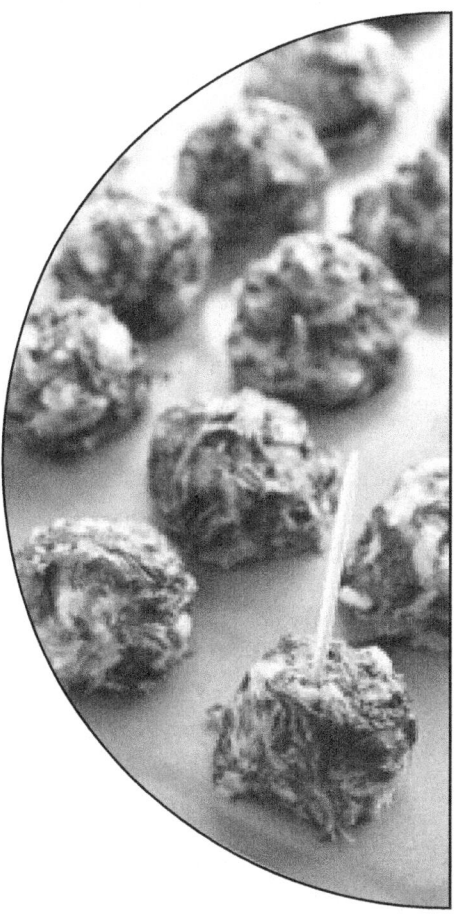

CHEESE & CHICKEN SANDWICH

Preparation Time: 15 minutes
Cooking Time: 5-7 minutes
Servings: 2

INGREDIENTS

- 1/3 cup of chicken, cooked and shredded
- 2 mozzarella slices
- 1 hamburger bun
- ¼ cup of cabbage, shredded
- 1 teaspoon of mayonnaise
- 2 teaspoon of butter
- 1 teaspoon of olive oil
- ½ teaspoon of balsamic vinegar
- 1/4 teaspoon of smoked paprika
- ¼ teaspoon of black pepper
- ¼ teaspoon of garlic powder
- Pinch of salt

DIRECTIONS

1. Preheat your Air Fryer at 370 °F.
2. Apply some butter to the outside of the hamburger bun with a brush.
3. In a bowl, coat the chicken with garlic powder, salt, pepper, and paprika.
4. In a separate bowl, stir together the mayonnaise, olive oil, cabbage, and balsamic vinegar to make coleslaw.
5. Slice the bun in two. Start building the sandwich, starting with the chicken, followed by the mozzarella, the coleslaw, and finally the top bun.
6. Transfer the sandwich to the fryer and cook for 5 – 7 minutes.

NUTRITION

- Calories: 314
- Fat: 11.5 g
- Fiber: 3.4 g
- Carbs: 11.5 g
- Protein: 5.6 g

BACON & HORSERADISH CREAM

Preparation Time: 1 hour 40 minutes
Cooking Time: 1 hour 40 minutes
Servings: 2

INGREDIENTS

- ½ lb. of thick cut bacon, diced
- 2 tablespoon of butter
- 2 shallots, sliced
- ½ cup of milk
- 1 ½ lb. of Brussels sprouts, halved
- 2 tablespoon of almond flour
- 1 cup of heavy cream
- 2 tablespoon of prepared horseradish
- ½ tablespoon of fresh thyme leaves
- 1/8 teaspoon of ground nutmeg
- 1 tablespoon of olive oil
- ½ teaspoon of sea salt
- Ground black pepper to taste
- ½ cup of water

DIRECTIONS

1. Preheat your Air Fryer at 400 °F.
2. Coat the Brussels sprouts with olive oil and sprinkle some salt and pepper on top. Transfer to the fryer and cook for a half-hour. Give them a good stir at the halfway point, then take them out of the fryer and set to the side.
3. Put the bacon in the fryer's basket and pour the water into the drawer underneath to catch the fat. Cook for 10 minutes, stirring 2 or 3 times throughout the cooking time.
4. When 10 minutes are up, add in the shallots. Cook for a further 10 – 15 minutes, making sure the shallots soften up and the bacon turns brown. Add some more pepper and remove. Leave to drain on some paper towels.
5. Melt the butter over the stove or in the microwave before adding in the flour and mixing with a whisk. Slowly add in the heavy cream and milk, and continue to whisk for another 3 – 5 minutes, making sure the mixture thickens.
6. Add the horseradish, thyme, salt, and nutmeg, and stir well once more.
7. Take a 9" x 13" baking dish and grease it with oil. Preheat your oven to 350 °F.
8. Put the Brussels sprouts in the baking dish and spread them across the base. Pour over the cream sauce and then top with a layer of bacon and shallots.
9. Cook in the oven for a half-hour and enjoy.

NUTRITION

- Calories: 346
- Fat: 11.5 g
- Fiber: 3.4 g
- Carbs: 11.5 g
- Protein: 5.6 g

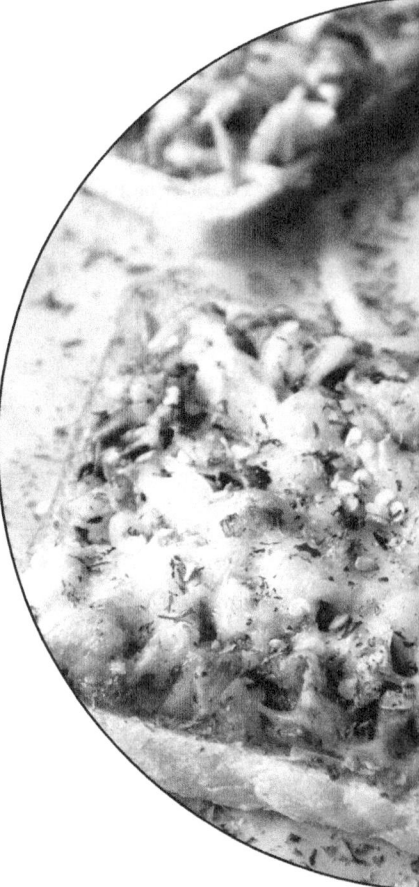

VEGETABLE TOAST

Preparation Time: 25 minutes
Cooking Time: 15 minutes
Servings: 2

INGREDIENTS

- 4 slices of bread
- 1 red bell pepper, cut into strips
- 1 cup of a sliced button or cremini mushrooms
- 1 small yellow squash, sliced
- 2 green onions, sliced
- 1 tablespoon of olive oil
- 2 tablespoons of softened butter
- ½ cup of soft goat cheese

DIRECTIONS

1. Drizzle the Air Fryer with olive oil and preheat to 350 °F.
2. Put the red pepper, green onions, mushrooms, and squash inside the fryer and give them a stir and cook for 7 minutes, shaking the basket once throughout the cooking time. Ensure the vegetables become tender.
3. Remove the vegetables and set them aside.
4. Spread some butter on the slices of bread and transfer to the Air Fryer, butter side-up. Brown for 2 to 4 minutes.
5. Remove the toast from the fryer and top with goat cheese and vegetables. Serve warm.

NUTRITION

- Calories: 246
- Fat: 11.5 g
- Fiber: 3.4 g
- Carbs: 11.5 g
- Protein: 5.6 g

CINNAMON TOASTS

Preparation Time: 15 minutes
Cooking Time: 5 minutes
Servings: 2

INGREDIENTS

- 10 bread slices
- 1 pack salted butter
- 4 tablespoons of stevia
- 2 teaspoon of ground cinnamon
- ½ teaspoon of vanilla extract

DIRECTIONS

1. In a bowl, combine the butter, cinnamon, stevia, and vanilla extract. Spread onto the slices of bread.
2. Set your Air Fryer to 380 °F. When warmed up, put the bread inside the fryer and cook for 4– 5 minutes.

NUTRITION

- Calories: 346
- Fat: 11.5 g
- Fiber: 3.4 g
- Carbs: 11.5 g
- Protein: 5.6 g

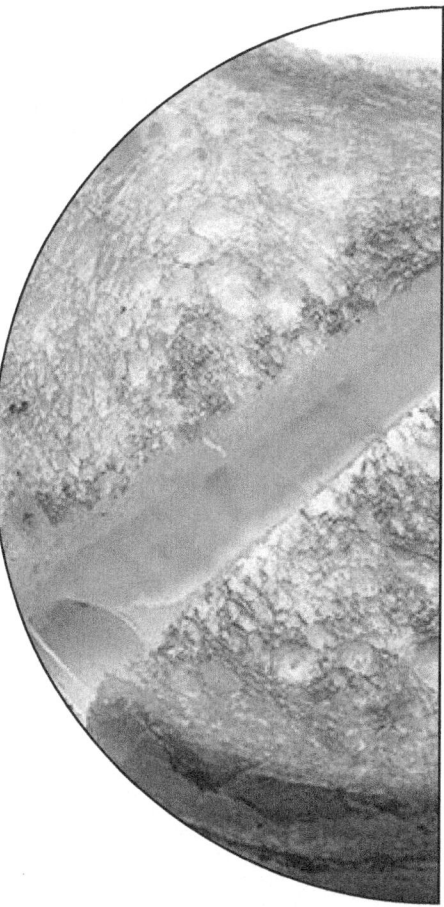

TOASTED CHEESE

Preparation Time: 20 minutes
Cooking Time: 5 minutes
Servings: 2

INGREDIENTS

- 2 slices of bread
- 4 oz. of cheese, grated
- A small amount of butter

DIRECTIONS

1. Grill the bread in the toaster.
2. Butter the toast and top with the grated cheese.
3. Set your Air Fryer to 350 °F and allow it to warm.
4. Put the toast slices inside the fryer and cook for 4 - 6 minutes.
5. Serve and enjoy!

NUTRITION

- Calories: 290
- Fat: 11.5 g
- Fiber: 3.4 g
- Carbs: 11.5 g
- Protein: 5.6 g

PEANUT BUTTER BREAD

Preparation Time: 15 minutes
Cooking Time: 5 minutes
Servings: 2

INGREDIENTS

- 1 tablespoon of oil
- 2 tablespoons of peanut butter
- 4 slices of bread
- 1 banana, sliced

DIRECTIONS

1. Spread the peanut butter on top of each slice of bread, then arrange the banana slices on top. Sandwich 2 slices together, then the other two.
2. Oil the inside of the Air Fryer and cook the bread for 5 minutes at 300 °F.

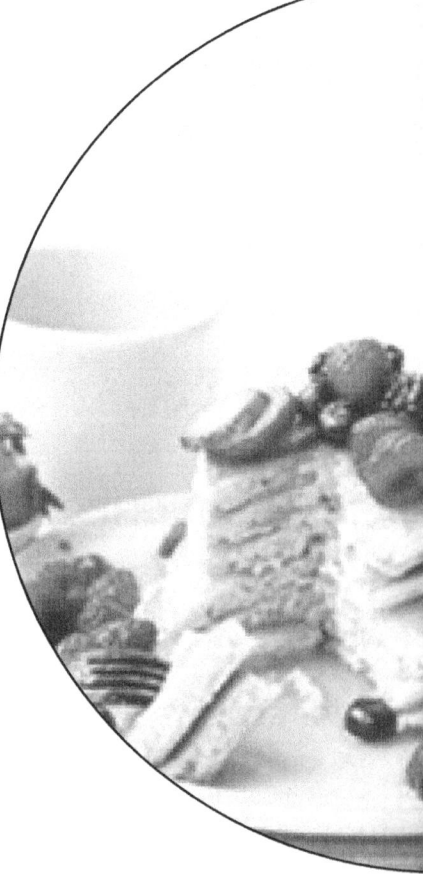

EASY BLENDER PANCAKES

Preparation Time: 25 minutes
Cooking Time: 15 minutes
Servings: 2

INGREDIENTS

- 2 eggs
- 2 oz. of cream cheese
- 1 scoop Isopure Protein Powder
- 1 pinch of salt
- 1 dash of cinnamon

DIRECTIONS

1. Mix the eggs with cream cheese, protein powder, salt, and cinnamon in a bowl.
2. Transfer to a blender and blend until smooth.
3. Heat a nonstick pan and pour a quarter of the mixture.
4. Cook for about 2 minutes on each side and dish out.
5. Repeat with the remaining mixture and dish out in a platter to serve warm.

THREE BEANS MIX

Preparation Time: 10 minutes
Cooking Time: 0 minutes
Servings: 2

INGREDIENTS

- 15 ounces canned kidney beans, no-salt-added, drained and rinsed
- 15 ounces canned garbanzo beans, no-salt-added and drained
- 15 ounces canned pinto beans, no-salt-added and drained
- 3 tablespoons balsamic vinegar
- 2 tablespoons olive oil
- 2 teaspoon Italian seasoning
- 2 teaspoons garlic powder
- 1 teaspoon onion powder

DIRECTIONS

1. In a large salad bowl, combine the beans with vinegar, oil, seasoning, garlic powder, and onion powder, toss, divide between plates and serve as a side dish.
2. Enjoy!

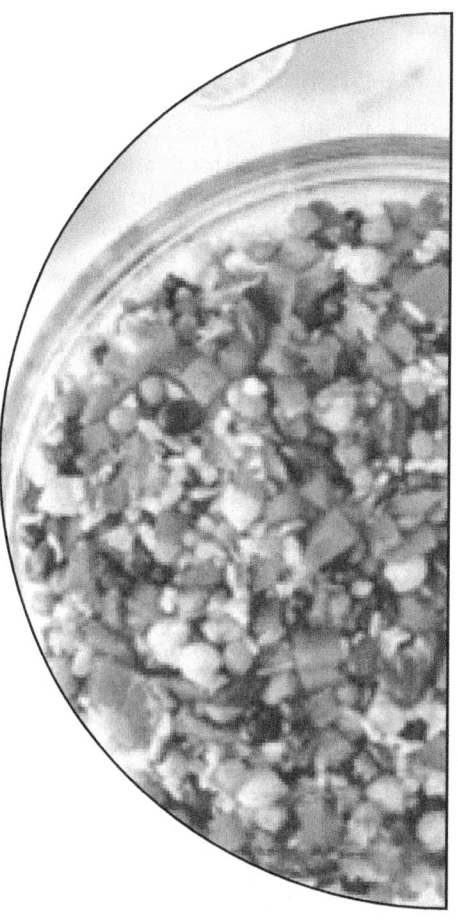

CREAMY CUCUMBER MIX

Preparation Time: 10 minutes
Cooking Time: 0 minutes
Servings: 2

INGREDIENTS

- 1 big cucumber, peeled and chopped
- 1 small red onion, chopped
- 4 tablespoons of non-fat yogurt
- 1 teaspoon of balsamic vinegar

DIRECTIONS

1. In a bowl, mix the onion with cucumber, yogurt, and vinegar, toss, divide between plates and serve as a side dish.
2. Enjoy!

BELL PEPPERS MIX

Preparation Time: 10 minutes
Cooking Time: 10 minutes
Servings: 2

INGREDIENTS

- 1 tablespoon olive oil
- 2 teaspoons garlic powder
- 2 red bell peppers, chopped
- 2 yellow bell peppers, chopped
- 2 orange bell peppers, chopped
- Black pepper to the taste

DIRECTIONS

1. Heat up a pan with the oil over medium-high heat, add all the bell peppers, stir and cook for 5 minutes.
2. Add garlic powder and black pepper, stir, cook for 5 minutes, divide between plates and serve as a side dish.
3. Enjoy!

NUTRITION

- Calories: 145
- Fat: 3 g
- Fiber: 5 g
- Carbs: 5 g
- Protein: 8 g

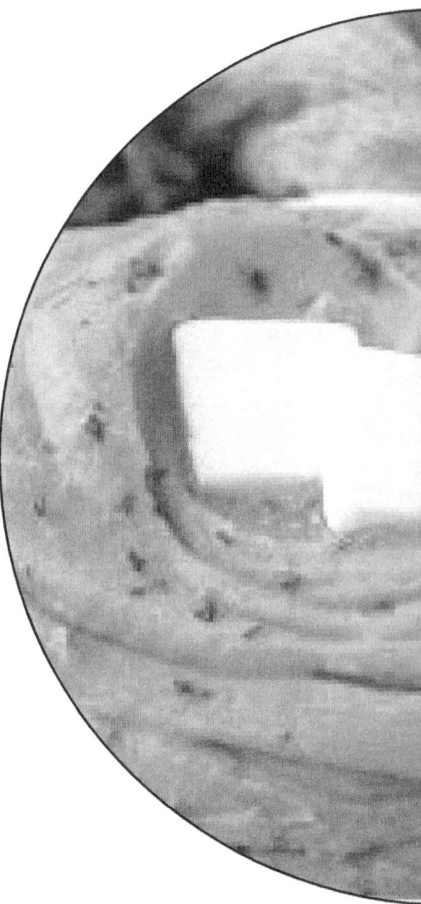

SWEET POTATO MASH

Preparation Time: 10 minutes
Cooking Time: 1 hour
Servings: 2

INGREDIENTS

- ¼ cup of olive oil
- 3 pounds of sweet potatoes
- Black pepper to the taste

DIRECTIONS

1. Arrange the sweet potatoes on a lined baking sheet, introduce in the oven, bake at 375 ° F for 1 hour, cool them down, peel, mash them, and put them in a bowl.
2. Add black pepper and the oil, whisk well. Divide between plates and serve as a side dish.
3. Enjoy!

NUTRITION

- Calories: 140
- Fat: 1 g
- Fiber: 4 g
- Carbs: 6 g
- Protein: 4 g

BOK CHOY MIX

Preparation Time: 10 minutes
Cooking Time: 15 minutes
Servings: 2

INGREDIENTS

- 2 tablespoons of olive oil
- 3 tablespoons of coconut aminos
- 1-inch ginger, grated
- A pinch of red pepper flakes
- 4 bok choy heads, cut into quarters
- 2 garlic cloves, minced
- 1 tablespoon of sesame seeds, toasted

DIRECTIONS

1. Heat a pan with the olive oil over medium heat, add coconut aminos, garlic, pepper flakes, ginger, stir, and cook for 3-4 minutes.
2. Add the bok choy and the sesame seeds, toss, cook for 5 minutes more, divide between plates and serve as a side dish.
3. Enjoy!

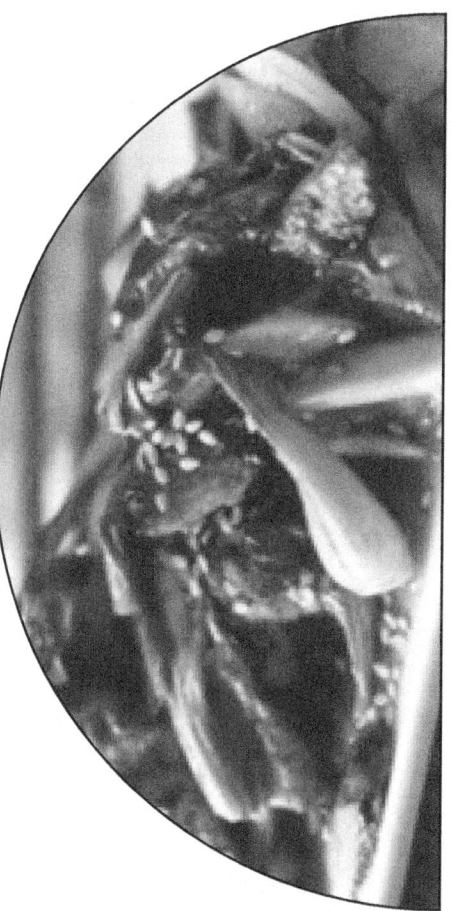

FLAVORED TURNIPS MIX

Preparation Time: 10 minutes
Cooking Time: 15 minutes
Servings: 2

INGREDIENTS

- 1 tablespoon of lemon juice
- Zest of 2 oranges, grated
- 16 ounces of turnips, sliced
- 3 tablespoons of olive oil
- 1 tablespoon of rosemary, chopped
- Black pepper to the taste

DIRECTIONS

1. Heat a pan with the oil over medium-high heat, add turnips, stir and cook for 5 minutes.
2. Add the lemon juice, black pepper, orange zest, and rosemary, stir, cook for 10 minutes more, divide between plates, and serve as a side dish.
3. Enjoy!

LEMONY FENNEL MIX

Preparation Time: 10 minutes
Cooking Time: 0 minutes
Servings: 2

INGREDIENTS

- 3 tablespoons lemon juice
- 1 pound fennel, chopped
- 2 tablespoons olive oil
- A pinch of black pepper

DIRECTIONS

1. In a salad bowl, mix fennel with and black pepper, oil, and lemon juice, toss well, divide between plates and serve as a side dish.
2. Enjoy!

NUTRITION

- Calories: 130
- Fat: 1 g
- Fiber: 1 g
- Carbs: 7 g
- Protein: 7 g

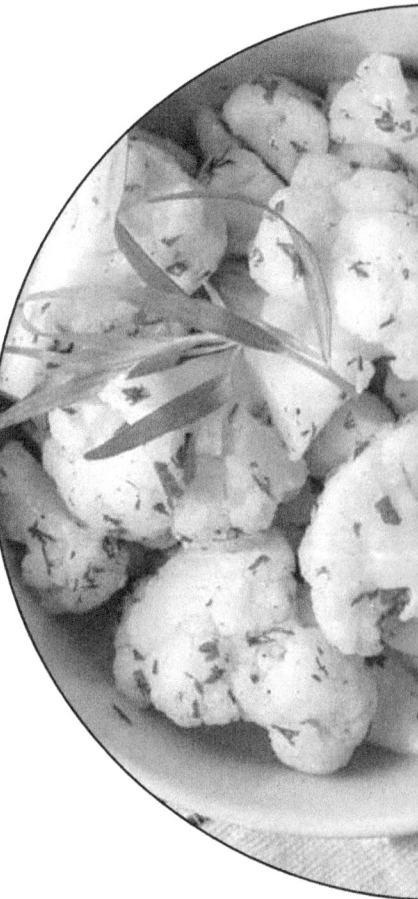

SIMPLE CAULIFLOWER MIX

Preparation Time: 10 minutes
Cooking Time: 35 minutes
Servings: 2

INGREDIENTS

- 6 cups of cauliflower florets
- 2 teaspoons of sweet paprika
- 2 cups of chicken stock
- ¼ cup of avocado oil
- Black pepper to the taste

DIRECTIONS

1. In a baking dish, combine the cauliflower with stock, oil, black pepper, and paprika, toss, introduce in the oven and bake at 375 ° F for 35 minutes.
2. Divide between plates and serve as a side dish.
3. Enjoy!

NUTRITION

- Calories: 180
- Fat: 3 g
- Fiber: 2 g
- Carbs: 46 g
- Protein: 6 g

BROCCOLI MIX

Preparation Time: 10 minutes
Cooking Time: 3 hours
Servings: 2

INGREDIENTS

- 6 cups of broccoli florets
- 10 ounces of tomato sauce, sodium-free
- 1 and ½ cups of low-fat cheddar cheese, shredded
- ½ teaspoon of cider vinegar
- ¼ cup of yellow onion, chopped
- A pinch of black pepper
- 2 tablespoons of olive oil

DIRECTIONS

1. Grease your slow cooker with the oil, add broccoli, tomato sauce, cider vinegar, onion, and black pepper, cover, and cook on High for 2 hours and 30 minutes.
2. Sprinkle the cheese all over, cover, cook on High for 30 minutes more, divide between plates and serve as a side dish.
3. Enjoy!

NUTRITION

- Calories: 160
- Fat: 6 g
- Fiber: 4 g
- Carbs: 11 g
- Protein: 6 g

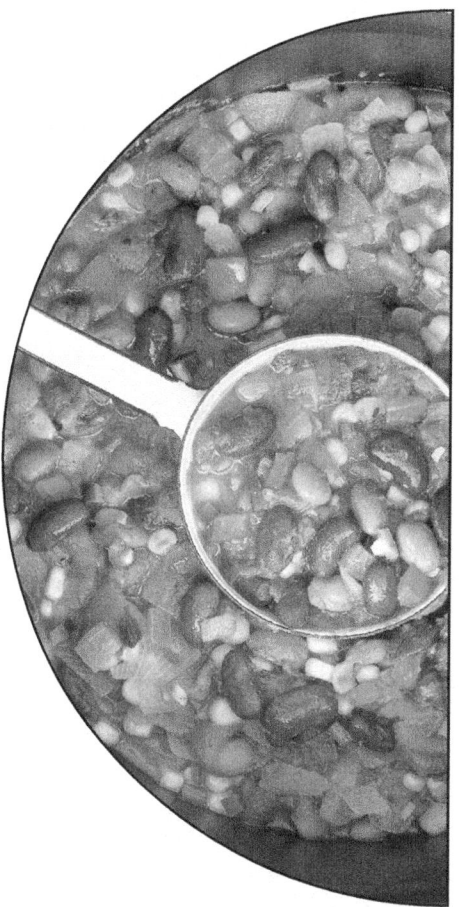

TASTY BEAN SIDE DISH

Preparation Time: 10 minutes
Cooking Time: 5 hours
Servings: 2

INGREDIENTS

- 1 and ½ cups of tomato sauce, salt-free
- 1 yellow onion, chopped
- 2 celery ribs, chopped
- 1 sweet red pepper, chopped
- 1 green bell pepper, chopped
- ½ cup of water
- 2 bay leaves
- 1 teaspoon of ground mustard
- 1 tablespoon of cider vinegar
- 16 ounces of canned kidney beans, no-salt-added, drained and rinsed
- 16 ounces of canned black-eyed peas, no-salt-added, drained and rinsed
- 15 ounces of corn
- 15 ounces of canned lima beans, no-salt-added, drained and rinsed
- 15 ounces of canned black beans, no-salt-added, drained and rinsed

DIRECTIONS

1. In your slow cooker, mix the tomato sauce with the onion, celery, red pepper, green bell pepper, water, bay leaves, mustard, vinegar, kidney beans, black-eyed peas, corn, lima beans, and black beans, cover and cook on Low for 5 hours.
2. Discard the bay leaves, divide the whole mix between plates, and serve.
3. Enjoy!

NUTRITION

- Calories: 211
- Fat: 4 g
- Fiber: 8 g
- Carbs: 20 g
- Protein: 7 g

EASY GREEN BEANS

Preparation Time: 10 minutes
Cooking Time: 2 hours
Servings: 2

INGREDIENTS

- 16 ounces of green beans
- 3 tablespoons of olive oil
- ½ cup of coconut sugar
- 1 teaspoon of low-sodium soy sauce
- ½ teaspoon of garlic powder

DIRECTIONS

1. In your slow cooker, mix the green beans with the oil, sugar, soy sauce, and garlic powder, cover, and cook on Low for 2 hours.
2. Toss the beans, divide them between plates and serve as a side dish.
3. Enjoy!

NUTRITION

- Calories: 142
- Fat: 7 g
- Fiber: 4 g
- Carbs: 15 g
- Protein: 3 g

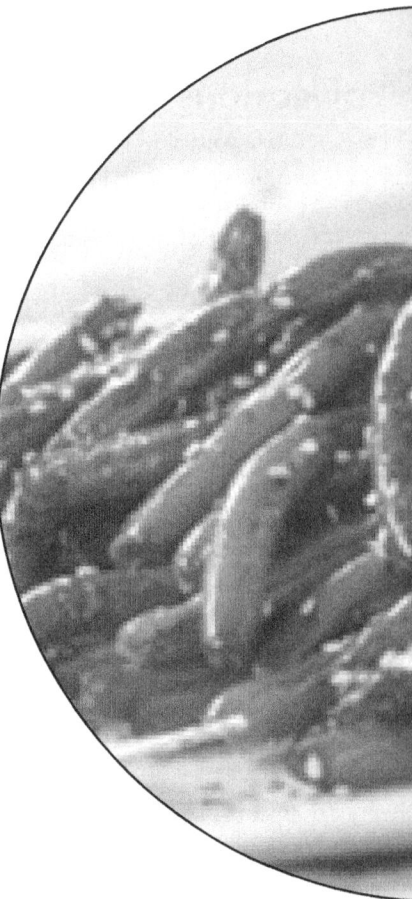

CREAMY CORN

Preparation Time: 10 minutes
Cooking Time: 4 hours
Servings: 2

INGREDIENTS

- 10 cups of corn
- 20 ounces of fat-free cream cheese
- ½ cup of fat-free milk
- ½ cup of low-fat butter
- A pinch of black pepper
- 2 tablespoons of green onions, chopped

DIRECTIONS

1. In your slow cooker, mix the corn with cream cheese, milk, butter, black pepper, and onions, toss, cover, and cook on Low for 4 hours.
2. Toss one more time, divide between plates and serve as a side dish.
3. Enjoy!

NUTRITION

- Calories: 256
- Fat: 11 g
- Fiber: 2 g
- Carbs: 17 g
- Protein: 5 g

LASSIC PEAS AND CARROTS

Preparation Time: 10 minutes
Cooking Time: 5 hours
Servings: 2

INGREDIENTS

- 1 pound of carrots, sliced
- ¼ cup of water
- 1 yellow onion, chopped
- 2 tablespoons of olive oil
- 2 tablespoons of stevia
- 4 garlic cloves, minced
- 1 teaspoon of marjoram, dried
- A pinch of white pepper
- 16 ounces of peas

DIRECTIONS

1. In your slow cooker, mix the carrots with water, onion, oil, stevia, garlic, marjoram, white pepper, and peas, toss, cover, and cook on High for 5 hours.
2. Divide between plates and serve as a side dish.
3. Enjoy!

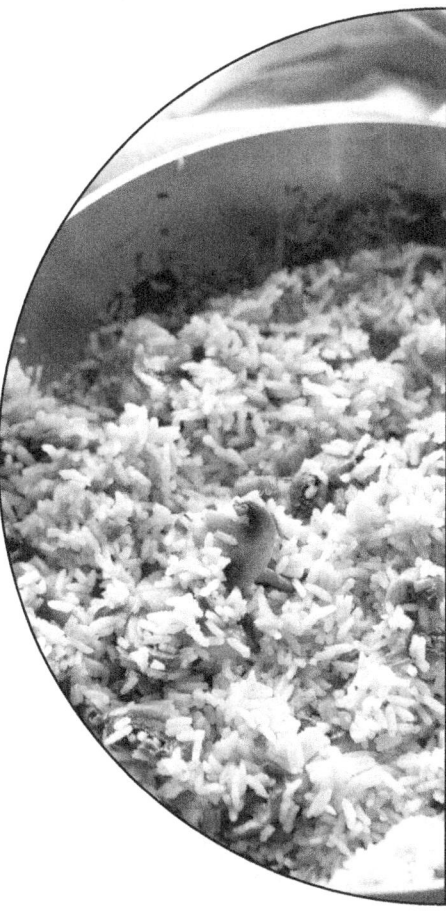

MUSHROOM PILAF

Preparation Time: 10 minutes
Cooking Time: 3 hours
Servings: 2

INGREDIENTS

- 1 cup of wild rice
- 2 garlic cloves, minced
- 6 green onions, chopped
- 2 tablespoons of olive oil
- ½ pound of baby Bella mushrooms
- 2 cups of water

DIRECTIONS

1. In your slow cooker, mix the rice with garlic, onions, oil, mushrooms, and water, toss, cover, and cook on Low for 3 hours.
2. Stir the pilaf one more time, divide between plates and serve.
3. Enjoy!

BUTTERNUT MIX

Preparation Time: 10 minutes
Cooking Time: 4 hours
Servings: 2

INGREDIENTS

- 1 cup of carrots, chopped
- 1 tablespoon of olive oil
- 1 yellow onion, chopped
- ½ teaspoon of stevia
- 1 garlic clove, minced
- ½ teaspoon of curry powder
- ½ teaspoon of cinnamon powder
- ¼ teaspoon of ginger, grated
- 1 butternut squash, cubed
- 2 and ½ cups of low-sodium veggie stock
- ¾ cup of coconut milk

DIRECTIONS

1. Heat a pan with the oil over medium-high heat, add the oil, onion, garlic, stevia, carrots, curry powder, cinnamon, and ginger, stir, cook for 5 minutes and transfer to your slow cooker.
2. Add the squash, stock, and coconut milk. Stir, cover, and cook on Low for 4 hours.
3. Divide the butternut mix between plates and serve as a side dish.
4. Enjoy!

NUTRITION

- Calories: 200
- Fat: 4 g
- Fiber: 4 g
- Carbs: 17 g
- Protein: 3 g

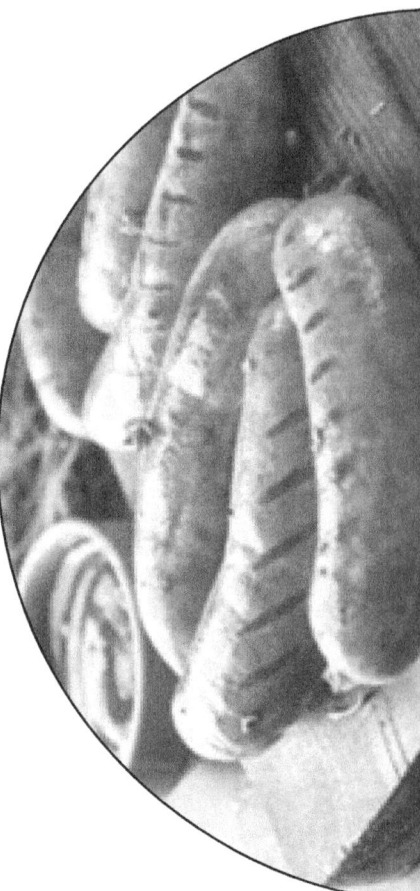

SAUSAGE SIDE DISH

Preparation Time: 10 minutes
Cooking Time: 2 hours
Servings: 2

INGREDIENTS

- 1 pound of no-sugar, beef sausage, chopped
- 2 tablespoons of olive oil
- ½ pound of mushrooms, chopped
- 6 celery ribs, chopped
- 2 yellow onions, chopped
- 2 garlic cloves, minced
- 1 tablespoon of sage, dried
- 1 cup of low-sodium veggie stock
- 1 cup of cranberries, dried
- ½ cup of sunflower seeds, peeled
- 1 whole-wheat bread loaf, cubed

DIRECTIONS

1. Heat a pan with the oil over medium-high heat, add beef, stir and brown for a few minutes.
2. Add the mushrooms, onion, celery, garlic, and sage, stir, cook for a few more minutes and transfer to your slow cooker.
3. Add the stock, cranberries, sunflower seeds, and bread cubes. Cover, and cook on High for 2 hours.
4. Stir the whole mix, divide between plates and serve as a side dish.
5. Enjoy!

NUTRITION

- Calories: 200
- Fat: 3 g
- Fiber: 6 g
- Carbs: 13 g
- Protein: 4 g

EASY POTATOES MIX

Preparation Time: 10 minutes
Cooking Time: 6 hours
Servings: 2

INGREDIENTS

- 16 baby red potatoes, halved
- 1 carrot, sliced
- 1 celery rib, chopped
- ¼ cup of yellow onion, chopped
- 2 cups of low-sodium chicken stock
- 1 tablespoon of parsley, chopped
- A pinch of black pepper
- 1 garlic clove minced
- 2 tablespoons of olive oil

DIRECTIONS

1. In your slow cooker, mix the potatoes with the carrot, celery, onion, stock, parsley, garlic, oil, and black pepper, toss, cover, and cook on Low for 6 hours.
2. Divide between plates and serve as a side dish.
3. Enjoy!

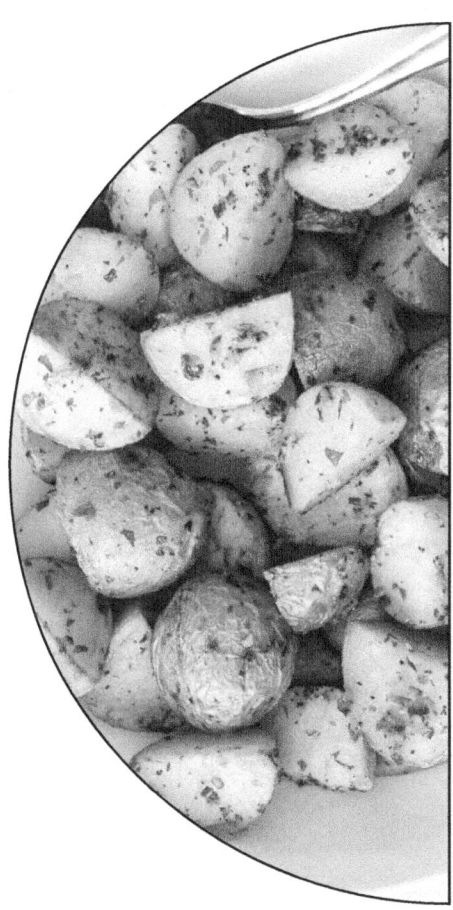

BLACK-EYED PEAS MIX

Preparation Time: 10 minutes
Cooking Time: 5 hours
Servings: 2

INGREDIENTS
- 17 ounces of black-eyed peas
- ½ cup of sausage, chopped
- 1 yellow onion, chopped
- 1 sweet red pepper, chopped
- 1 jalapeno, chopped
- 2 garlic cloves minced
- ½ teaspoon of cumin, ground
- A pinch of black pepper
- 6 cups of water
- 2 tablespoons of cilantro, chopped

DIRECTIONS

1. In your slow cooker, mix the peas with the sausage, onion, red pepper, jalapeno, garlic, cumin, black pepper, water, cilantro, cover, and cook on Low for 5 hours.
2. Divide between plates and serve as a side dish.
3. Enjoy!

CHAPTER 3.
SEAFOOD

STEAMED SALMON TERIYAKI

Preparation Time: 10 minutes
Cooking Time: 15 minutes
Servings: 2

INGREDIENTS

- 3 green onions, minced
- 2 packet of Stevia
- 1 tablespoon of freshly grated ginger
- 1 clove of garlic, minced
- 2 teaspoon of sesame seeds
- 1 tablespoon of sesame oil
- ¼ cup of mirin
- 2 tablespoons of low sodium soy sauce
- 1/2-lb. of salmon filet

DIRECTIONS

1. Place a large saucepan on the medium-high fire. Place a trivet inside the saucepan and fill the pan halfway with water. Cover and bring to a boil.
2. Meanwhile, in a heatproof dish that fits inside the saucepan, mix well stevia, ginger, garlic, oil, mirin, and soy sauce. Add salmon and cover well with the sauce.
3. Top the salmon with sesame seeds and green onions. Cover dish with foil.
4. Place on top of the trivet. Cover and steam for 15 minutes.
5. Let it rest for 5 minutes in the pan.
6. Serve and enjoy.

NUTRITION

- Calories: 242.7
- Carbs: 1.2 g
- Protein: 35.4 g
- Fat 10.7 g
- Saturated Fat: 2.1 g
- Sodium: 285 mg

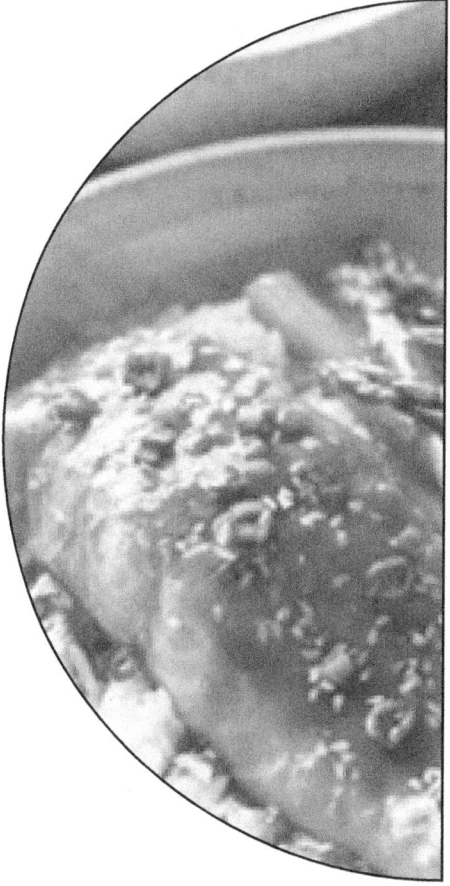

EASY STEAMED ALASKAN COD

Preparation Time: 10 minutes
Cooking Time: 15 minutes
Servings: 2

INGREDIENTS

- 2 tablespoon of butter
- Pepper to taste
- 1 cup of cherry tomatoes, halved
- 1 large Wild Alaskan cod filet, cut into 3 smaller pieces

DIRECTIONS

1. Place a large saucepan on the medium-high fire. Place a trivet inside the saucepan and fill the pan halfway with water. Cover and bring to a boil.
2. Meanwhile, in a heatproof dish that fits inside the saucepan, add all ingredients.
3. Cover dish with a foil. Place on trivet and steam for 15 minutes.
4. Serve and enjoy.

NUTRITION

- Calories: 132.9
- Carbs: 1.9 g
- Protein: 12.2 g
- Fat 8.5 g
- Saturated Fat: 4.9 g
- Sodium: 296 mg

DILL AND LEMON COD PACKETS

Preparation Time: 10 minutes
Cooking Time: 10 minutes
Servings: 2

INGREDIENTS

- 2 teaspoon of olive oil, divided
- 4 slices of lemon, divided
- 2 sprigs of fresh dill, divided
- ½ teaspoon of garlic powder, divided
- Pepper to taste
- 1/2-lb. of cod filets

DIRECTIONS

1. Place a large saucepan on the medium-high fire. Place a trivet inside the saucepan and fill the pan halfway with water. Cover and bring to a boil.
2. Cut 2 pieces of 15-inch length foil.
3. In one foil, place one filet in the middle. Season with pepper to taste. Sprinkle ¼ teaspoon of garlic. Add a teaspoon of oil on top of the filet. Top with 2 slices of lemon and a sprig of dill. Fold over the foil and seal the filet inside. Repeat the process for the remaining fish.
4. Place the packet on the trivet. Cover and steam for 10 minutes.
5. Serve and enjoy.

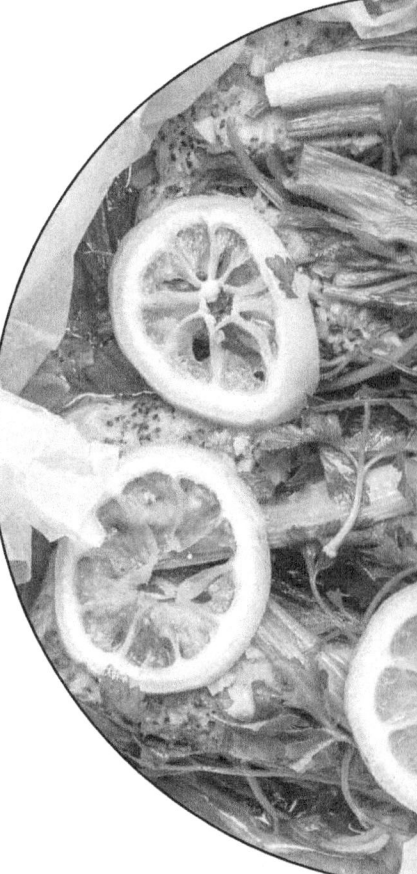

NUTRITION

- Calories: 164.8
- Carbs: 9.4 g
- Protein: 18.3 g
- Fat: 6 g
- Saturated Fat: 1 g
- Sodium: 347 mg

STEAMED FISH MEDITERRANEAN STYLE

Preparation Time: 10 minutes
Cooking Time: 15 minutes
Servings: 2

INGREDIENTS

- Pepper to taste
- 1 clove of garlic, smashed
- 2 teaspoon of olive oil
- 1 bunch of fresh thyme
- 2 tablespoons of pickled capers
- 1 cup of black salt-cured olives
- 1-lb. of cherry tomatoes halved
- 1 ½-lbs. of cod filets
- Capers and olives for garnish

DIRECTIONS

1. Place a large saucepan on a medium-high fire. Place a trivet inside the saucepan and fill the pan halfway with water. Cover and bring to a boil.
2. Meanwhile, in a heatproof dish that fits inside the saucepan, layer half of the halved cherry tomatoes. Season with pepper.
3. Add the filets on top of the tomatoes and season with pepper. Drizzle oil. Sprinkle 3/4s of thyme on top and the smashed garlic.
4. Cover the top of fish with the remaining cherry tomatoes plus the capers and olives then place the dish on the trivet. Cover the dish with foil.
5. Cover the pan and steam for 15 minutes.
6. Serve and enjoy.

NUTRITION

- Calories: 263.2
- Carbs: 21.8 g
- Protein: 27.8 g
- Fat 7.2 g
- Saturated Fat: 1.1 g
- Sodium: 264 mg

STEAMED VEGGIE AND LEMON PEPPER SALMON

Preparation Time: 10 minutes
Cooking Time: 15 minutes
Servings: 2

INGREDIENTS

- 1 carrot, peeled and julienned
- 1 red bell pepper, julienned
- 1 zucchini, julienned
- ½ lemon, sliced thinly
- 1 teaspoon of pepper
- ½ teaspoon of salt
- 1/2-lb. of salmon filet with skin on
- A dash of tarragon

DIRECTIONS

1. Place a large saucepan on the medium-high fire. Place a trivet inside the saucepan and fill the pan halfway with water. Cover and bring to a boil.
2. Meanwhile, in a heatproof dish that fits inside the saucepan, add the salmon with the skin side down. Season with pepper. Add slices of lemon on top.
3. Place the julienned vegetables on top of the salmon and season with tarragon. Cover dish with foil.
4. Cover pan and steam for 15 minutes.
5. Serve and enjoy.

NUTRITION

- Calories: 216.2
- Carbs: 4.1 g
- Protein: 35.1 g
- Fat: 6.6 g
- Saturated Fat: 1.5 g
- Sodium: 332 mg

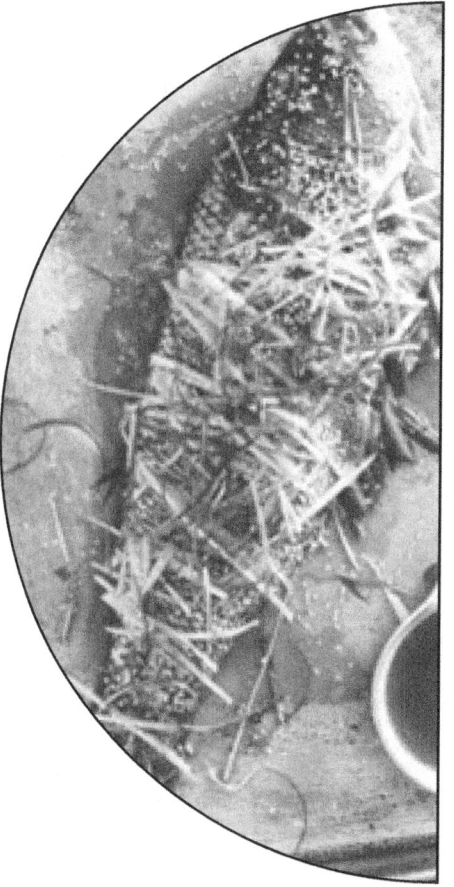

STEAMED FISH WITH SCALLIONS AND GINGER

Preparation Time: 10 minutes
Cooking Time: 15 minutes
Servings: 2

INGREDIENTS

- 1-lb. of Tilapia filets
- 1 teaspoon of garlic
- 1 teaspoon of minced ginger
- 2 tablespoon of rice wine
- 1 tablespoon of low sodium soy sauce

DIRECTIONS

1. In a heatproof dish that fits inside the saucepan, add garlic, minced ginger, rice wine, and soy sauce. Mix well. Add the Tilapia filet and marinate for half an hour while turning it over at a half time.
2. Place a large saucepan on the medium-high fire. Place a trivet inside the saucepan and fill the pan halfway with water. Cover and bring to a boil.
3. Cover the dish of fish with foil and place on trivet.
4. Cover the pan and steam for 15 minutes.
5. Serve and enjoy.

NUTRITION

- Calories: 219
- Carbs: 4.5 g
- Protein: 31.8 g
- Fat: 8.2 g
- Saturated Fat: 1.9 g
- Sodium: 252 mg

STEAMED TILAPIA WITH GREEN CHUTNEY

Cooking Time: 10 minutes
Preparation Time: 10 minutes
Servings: 2

INGREDIENTS

- 1-pound of tilapia fillets, divided into 3
- ½ cup of green commercial chutney

DIRECTIONS

1. Place a large saucepan on the medium-high fire. Place a trivet inside the saucepan and fill the pan halfway with water. Cover and bring to a boil.
2. Cut 3 pieces of 15-inch length foil.
3. In one foil, place 1 filet in the middle and 1/3 of chutney. Fold over the foil and seal the filet inside. Repeat the process for the remaining fish.
4. Place packet on a trivet. Cover and steam for 10 minutes.
5. Serve and enjoy.

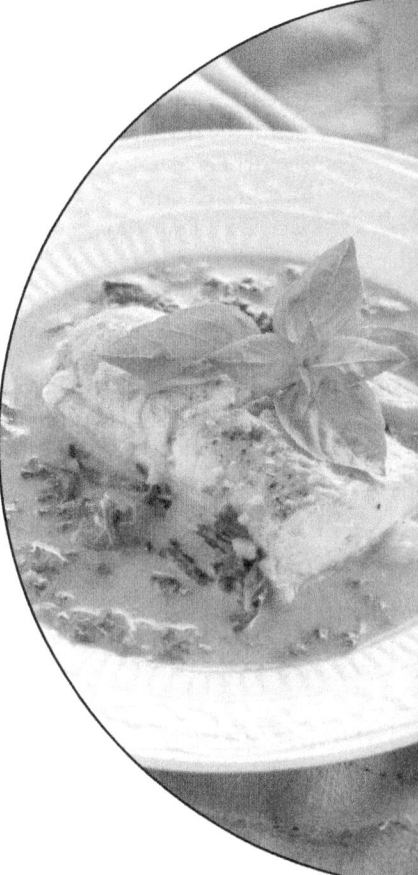

CREAMY HADDOCK WITH KALE

Cooking Time: 10 minutes
Preparation Time: 10 minutes
Servings: 2

INGREDIENTS

- 1 tablespoon of olive oil
- 1 onion, chopped
- 2 cloves of garlic, minced
- 2 cups of chicken broth
- 1 teaspoon of crushed red pepper flakes
- 1-pound of wild Haddock fillets
- ½ cup of heavy cream
- 1 tablespoon of basil
- 1 cup of kale leaves, chopped
- Pepper to taste

DIRECTIONS

1. Place a heavy bottomed pot on medium-high fire and heat pot for 3 minutes.
2. Once hot, add oil and stir around to coat the pot with oil.
3. Sauté the onion and garlic for 5 minutes.
4. Add the remaining ingredients, except for basil, and mix well.
5. Cover, bring to a boil, lower the fire to a simmer, and simmer for 5 minutes.
6. Serve and enjoy with a sprinkle of basil.

COCONUT CURRY SEA BASS

Preparation Time: 10 minutes
Cooking Time: 5 minutes
Servings: 2

INGREDIENTS

- 2 pcs. medium sized sea bass
- 1 can of coconut milk
- Juice of 1 lime, freshly squeezed
- 1 tablespoon of red curry paste
- 1 teaspoon of coconut aminos
- 1 teaspoon of honey
- 2 teaspoons of sriracha
- 2 cloves of garlic, minced
- 1 teaspoon of ground turmeric
- 1 tablespoon of curry powder
- ¼ cup of fresh cilantro
- Pepper

DIRECTIONS

1. Place a heavy bottomed pot on medium-high fire.
2. Mix in all the ingredients.
3. Cover, bring to a boil, lower the fire to a simmer, and simmer for 5 minutes.
4. Serve and enjoy.

NUTRITION

- Calories: 241.8
- Carbs: 12.8 g
- Protein: 3.1 g
- Fat: 19.8 g
- Saturated Fat: 17 g
- Sodium: 19 mg

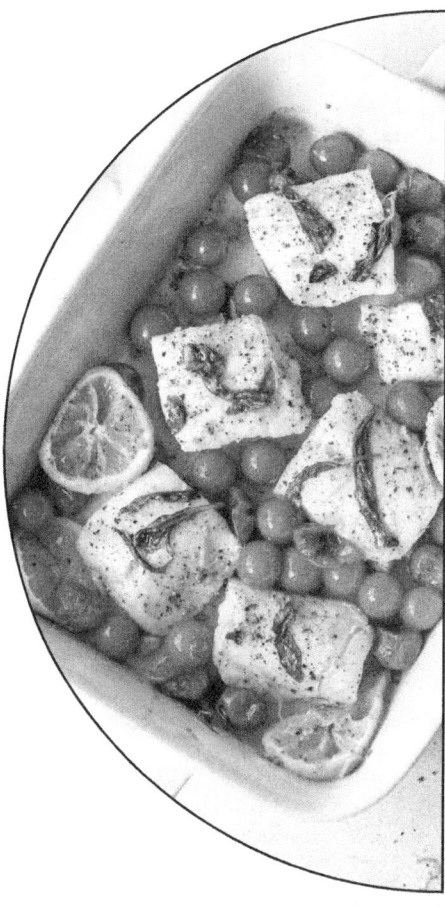

STEWED COD FILET WITH TOMATOES

Preparation Time: 10 minutes
Cooking Time: 15 minutes
Servings: 2

INGREDIENTS

- 1 tablespoon of olive oil
- 1 onion, sliced
- 1 ½ pound of fresh cod fillets
- Pepper
- 1 lemon juice, freshly squeezed
- 1 can of diced tomatoes

DIRECTIONS

1. Place a heavy bottomed pot on medium-high fire and heat pot for 3 minutes.
2. Once hot, add oil and stir around to coat the pot with oil.
3. Sauté the onion for 2 minutes. Stir in diced tomatoes and cook for 5 minutes.
4. Add the cod filet and season with pepper.
5. Cover, bring to a boil, lower the fire to a simmer, and simmer for 5 minutes.
6. Serve and enjoy with freshly squeezed lemon juice.

NUTRITION

- Calories: 106.4
- Carbs: 2.5 g
- Protein: 17.8 g
- Fat: 2.8 g
- Saturated Fat: 4 g
- Sodium: 38 1mg

LEMONY PARMESAN SHRIMPS

Preparation Time: 10 minutes
Cooking Time: 15 minutes
Servings: 2

INGREDIENTS

- 1 tablespoon of olive oil
- ½ cup of onion, chopped
- 3 cloves of garlic, minced
- 1-pound of shrimps, peeled and deveined
- ½ cup of parmesan cheese, low fat
- 1 cup of spinach, shredded
- ½ cup of chicken broth, low sodium
- ¼ cup of water
- Pepper

DIRECTIONS

1. Place a heavy bottomed pot on medium-high fire and heat pot for 3 minutes.
2. Once hot, add oil and stir around to coat the pot with oil.
3. Sauté the onion and garlic for 5 minutes. Stir in shrimps and cook for 2 minutes.
4. Add the remaining ingredients, except for the parmesan.
5. Cover, bring to a boil, lower the fire to a simmer, and simmer for 5 minutes.
6. Serve and enjoy with a sprinkle of parmesan.

NUTRITION

- Calories: 252.6
- Carbs: 5.4 g
- Protein: 33.9 g
- Fat: 10.6 g
- Saturated Fat: 3.2 g
- Sodium: 344 mg

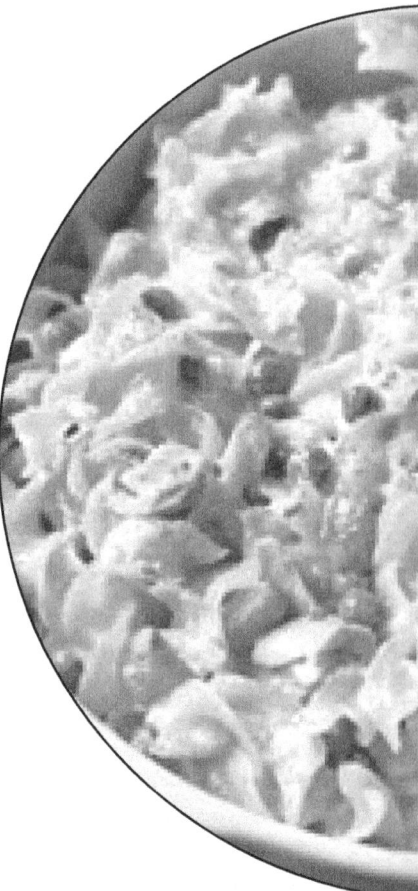

TUNA 'N CARROTS CASSEROLE

Preparation Time: 10 minutes
Cooking Time: 12 minutes
Servings: 2

INGREDIENTS

- 2 carrots, peeled and chopped
- ¼ cup of diced onions
- 1 cup of frozen peas
- ¾ cup of milk
- 2 cans of tuna in water, drained
- 1 can of cream of celery soup
- 1 tablespoon of olive oil
- ½ cup of water
- 2 eggs beaten
- Pepper

DIRECTIONS

1. Place a heavy bottomed pot on medium-high fire and heat pot for 3 minutes.
2. Once hot, add the oil and stir around to coat the pot with oil.
3. Sauté the onion and carrots for 3 minutes.
4. Add the remaining ingredients and mix well.
5. Bring to a boil while constantly stirring, cook until thickened around 5 minutes.
6. Serve and enjoy.

NUTRITION

- Calories: 281.3
- Carbs: 14.3 g
- Protein: 24.3 g
- Fat: 14.1 g
- Saturated Fat: 3.7 g
- Sodium: 275 mg

SWEET-GINGER SCALLOPS

Preparation Time: 10 minutes
Cooking Time: 15 minutes
Servings: 2

INGREDIENTS

- 1-pound of sea scallops, shells removed
- ½ cup of coconut aminos
- 3 tablespoons of maple syrup
- ½ teaspoon of garlic powder
- ½ teaspoon of ground ginger

DIRECTIONS

1. In a heatproof dish that fits inside the saucepan, add all ingredients. Mix well.
2. Place a large saucepan on medium-high fire. Place a trivet inside the saucepan and fill the pan halfway with water. Cover and bring to a boil.
3. Cover dish of scallops with foil and place on trivet.
4. Cover pan and steam for 10 minutes. Let it rest in the pan for another 5 minutes.
5. Serve and enjoy.

NUTRITION

- Calories: 233.4
- Carbs: 23.7 g
- Protein: 31.5 g
- Fat: 1.4 g
- Saturated Fat: 4 g
- Sodium: 153 mg

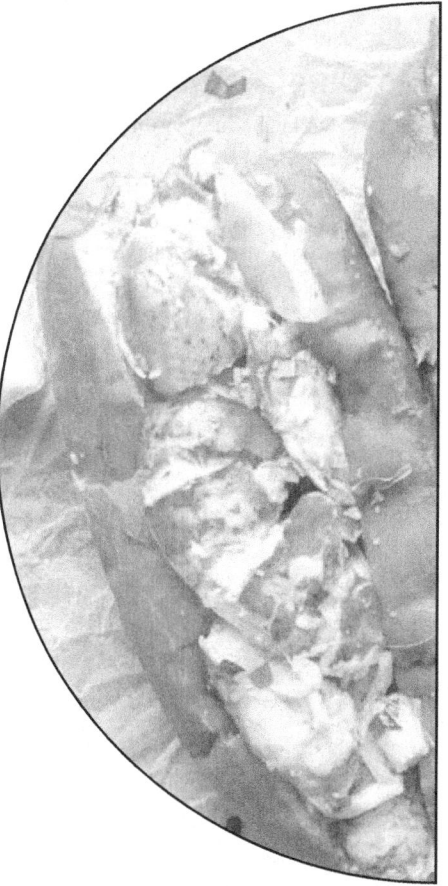

SAVORY LOBSTER ROLL

Preparation Time: 10 minutes
Cooking Time: 20 minutes
Servings: 2

INGREDIENTS

- 1 ½ cups of chicken broth, low sodium
- 2 teaspoon of old bay seasoning
- 2 pounds of lobster tails, raw and in the shell
- 1 lemon, halved
- 3 scallions, chopped
- 1 teaspoon of celery seeds

DIRECTIONS

1. Place a heavy bottomed pot on medium-high fire and add all the ingredients and ½ of the lemon.
2. Cover, bring to a boil, lower the fire to a simmer, and simmer for 15 minutes.
3. Let it rest for another 5 minutes.
4. Serve and enjoy with freshly squeezed lemon juice.

NUTRITION

- Calories: 209
- Carbs: 1.9 g
- Protein: 38.2 g
- Fat: 5.4 g
- Saturated Fat: 1.4 g
- Sodium: 288 mg

GARLIC 'N TOMATOES ON MUSSELS

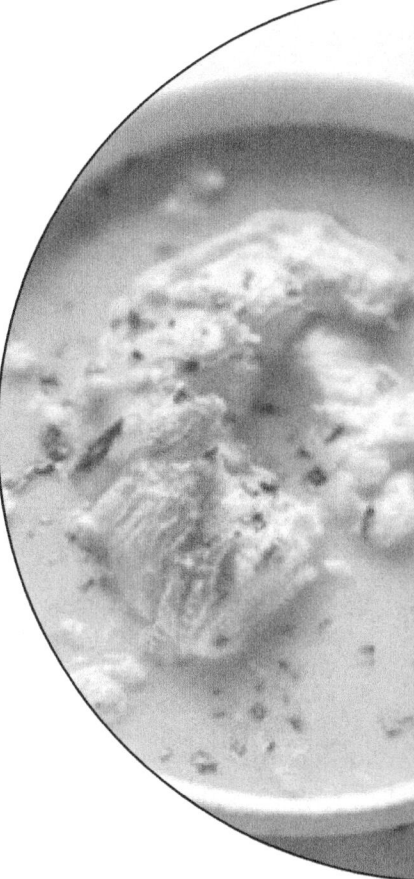

Preparation Time: 10 minutes
Cooking Time: 15 minutes
Servings: 2

INGREDIENTS

- ¼ cup of white wine
- ½ cup of water
- 3 Roma tomatoes, chopped
- 2 cloves of garlic, minced
- 1 bay leaf
- 2 pounds of mussels, scrubbed
- ½ cup of fresh parsley, chopped
- 1 tablespoon of oil
- Pepper

DIRECTIONS

1. Place a heavy bottomed pot on medium-high fire and heat pot for 3 minutes.
2. Once hot, add oil and stir around to coat the pot with oil.
3. Sauté the garlic, bay leaf, and tomatoes for 5 minutes.
4. Add the remaining ingredients, except for parsley and mussels. Mix well.
5. Add the mussels.
6. Cover and bring to a boil for 5 minutes.
7. Serve and enjoy with a sprinkle of parsley and discard any unopened mussels.

NUTRITION

- Calories: 172.8
- Carbs: 10.2 g
- Protein: 19.5 g
- Fat: 6 g
- Saturated Fat: 1.1 g
- Sodium: 261 mg

LOBSTER TARRAGON STEW

Preparation Time: 10 minutes
Cooking Time: 30 minutes
Servings: 2

INGREDIENTS

- 1 tablespoon of olive oil
- 2 onions, diced
- 2 cloves of garlic, minced
- 1 carrot, chopped
- 2 lobsters, shelled
- 1-pound of ripe tomatoes, chopped
- 2 tablespoons of tomato paste
- 1/3 clam juice
- 1 tablespoon of tarragon

DIRECTIONS

1. Place a heavy bottomed pot on medium-high fire and heat pot for 3 minutes.
2. Once hot, add oil and stir around to coat the pot with oil.
3. Sauté the onion, tomatoes, and garlic for 10 minutes.
4. Stir in tomato paste, clam juice, and carrot. Cook for 5 minutes.
5. Add lobsters and mix well.
6. Cover and simmer for 5 minutes.
7. Serve and enjoy with a sprinkle of tarragon.

NUTRITION

- Calories: 149.9
- Carbs: 13.3 g
- Protein: 14.5 g
- Fat: 4.3 g
- Saturated Fat: 1 g
- Sodium: 341 mg

EASY STEAMED CRAB LEGS

Preparation Time: 10 minutes
Cooking Time: 10 minutes
Servings: 2

INGREDIENTS

- 2 pounds of frozen crab legs
- 4 tablespoons of low fat butter
- 1 tablespoon of lemon juice, freshly squeezed

DIRECTIONS

1. Place a heavy bottomed pot on medium-high fire, fill with 5 cups water and bring to a boil.
2. Add the crab legs, cover, and steam for 10 minutes. Once done, turn off the fire and let it rest for 5 minutes.
3. Meanwhile, in a microwave-safe bowl, melt the butter. Once melted, add the lemon juice and mix well.
4. Serve the crab legs with the lemon-butter dip on the side.

NUTRITION

- Calories: 201.9
- Carbs: 2.2 g
- Protein: 44 g
- Fat: 1.9 g
- Saturated Fat: 3 g
- Sodium: 297 mg

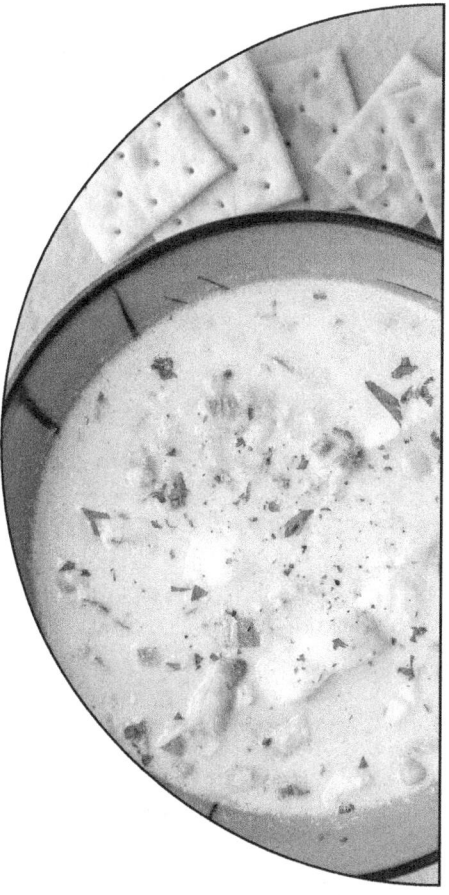

TASTY CORN AND CLAM STEW

Preparation Time: 10 minutes
Cooking Time: 25 minutes
Servings: 2

INGREDIENTS

- 1-lb. of clam
- 1 cup of frozen corn
- ½ cup of water
- 4 cloves of garlic
- 1 teaspoon of oil
- 1 teaspoon of celery seeds
- 1 teaspoon of Cajun seasoning

DIRECTIONS

1. Place a nonstick saucepan on medium-high fire and heat pot for 3 minutes.
2. Once hot, add oil and stir around to coat the pot with oil.
3. Sauté the garlic for a minute.
4. Add the remaining ingredients, except for the clams, and mix well. Cook for 3 minutes.
5. Stir in clams.
6. Cover, bring to a boil, lower the fire to a simmer, and simmer for 5 minutes.
7. Serve and enjoy. Discard any unopened clam.

NUTRITION

- Calories: 120
- Carbs: 23.2 g
- Protein: 2.3 g
- Fat: 2 g
- Saturated Fat: 2 g
- Sodium: 466 mg

SEAFOOD CURRY RECIPE FROM JAPAN

Preparation Time: 10 minutes
Cooking Time: 30 minutes
Servings: 2

INGREDIENTS

- 3 onions, chopped
- 2 cloves of garlic, minced
- 1-inch of ginger, grated
- 1 teaspoon of oil
- 3 cups of water
- 1 2-inch of long kombu or dried kelp
- 6 shiitake mushrooms, halved
- 12 manila clams, scrubbed
- 6 ounces of medium-sized shrimps, peeled and deveined
- 6 ounces of bay scallops
- 1 package of Japanese curry roux
- ¼ apple, sliced

DIRECTIONS

1. Place a heavy bottomed pot on medium-high fire and heat pot for 3 minutes.
2. Once hot, add oil and stir around to coat the pot with oil.
3. Sauté the onion, ginger, and garlic for 5 minutes.
4. Add the remaining ingredients and mix well.
5. Cover, bring to a boil, lower the fire to a simmer, and simmer for 5 minutes. Let it rest for 5 minutes.
6. Serve and enjoy. Discard any unopened clams.

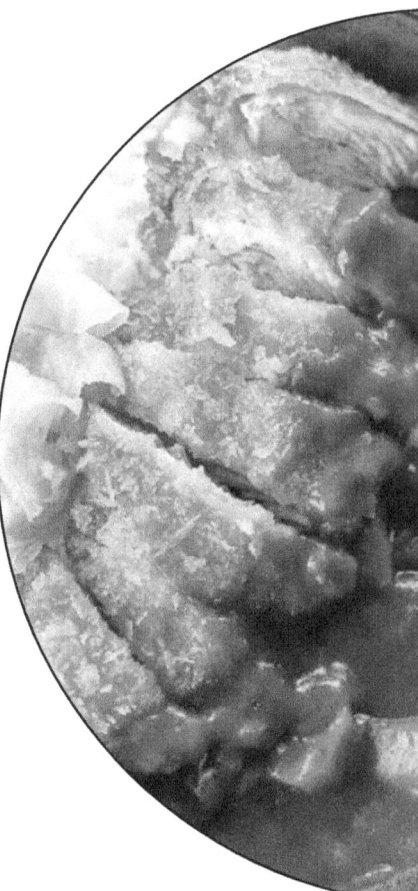

STEAMED ASPARAGUS AND SHRIMPS

Preparation Time: 10 minutes
Cooking Time: 25 minutes
Servings: 2

INGREDIENTS

- 1-pound of shrimps, peeled and deveined
- 1 bunch of asparagus, trimmed
- 1 teaspoon of oil
- ½ tablespoon of Cajun seasoning

DIRECTIONS

1. In a heatproof dish that fits inside the saucepan, add all the ingredients. Mix well.
2. Place a large saucepan on a medium-high fire. Place a trivet inside the saucepan and fill the pan halfway with water. Cover and bring to a boil.
3. Cover the dish with foil and place on trivet.
4. Cover the pan and steam for 10 minutes. Let it rest in the pan for another 5 minutes.
5. Serve and enjoy.

COCONUT MILK SAUCE OVER CRABS

Preparation Time: 10 minutes
Cooking Time: 20 minutes
Servings: 2

INGREDIENTS

- 2-pounds of crab quartered
- 1 can of coconut milk
- 1 lemongrass stalk
- 1 thumb-size ginger, sliced
- 1 onion, chopped
- 3 cloves of garlic, minced
- Pepper

DIRECTIONS

1. Place a heavy bottomed pot on medium-high fire and add all the ingredients.
2. Cover, bring to a boil, lower the fire to a simmer, and simmer for 10 minutes.
3. Serve and enjoy.

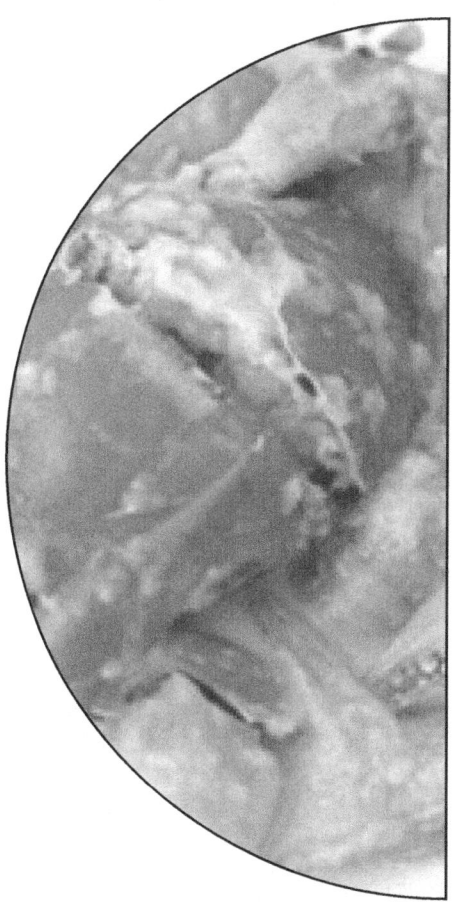

CAJUN SHRIMP BOIL

Preparation Time: 10 minutes
Cooking Time: 40 minutes
Servings: 2

INGREDIENTS

- 2 corn on the cobs, halved
- 1/2 kielbasa sausage, sliced into 2-inch pieces
- 1 cup of chicken broth, low sodium
- 1 tablespoon of old bay seasoning
- 1 teaspoon of celery seeds
- 4 garlic cloves, smashed
- 1 teaspoon of crushed red peppers
- 4 small potatoes, brushed and halved
- 1 onion, chopped
- 1-pound of shrimps
- 1 tablespoon of olive oil
- Pepper

DIRECTIONS

1. Place a heavy bottomed pot on medium-high fire and heat pot for 3 minutes.
2. Once hot, add the oil and stir around to coat the pot with oil.
3. Sauté the garlic, onion, potatoes, and sausage for 5 minutes.
4. Stir in the corn, broth, old bay, celery seeds, and red peppers. Cover and cook for 5 minutes.
5. Stir in the shrimps and cook for another 5 minutes.
6. Serve and enjoy.

SAUTÉED SAVORY SHRIMPS

Preparation Time: 10 minutes
Cooking Time: 15 minutes
Servings: 2

INGREDIENTS

- 2 pounds of shrimps, peeled and deveined
- 1 tablespoon of olive oil
- 4 cloves garlic, minced
- 2 cups of frozen sweet corn kernels
- ½ cup of chicken stock, low sodium
- 1 tablespoon of lemon juice
- Pepper
- 1 tablespoon of parsley for garnish

DIRECTIONS

1. Place a heavy bottomed pot on medium-high fire and heat pot for 3 minutes.
2. Once hot, add oil and stir around to coat the pot with oil.
3. Sauté the garlic and corn for 5 minutes.
4. Add the remaining ingredients and mix well.
5. Cover, bring to a boil, lower the fire to a simmer, and simmer for 5 minutes.
6. Serve and enjoy.

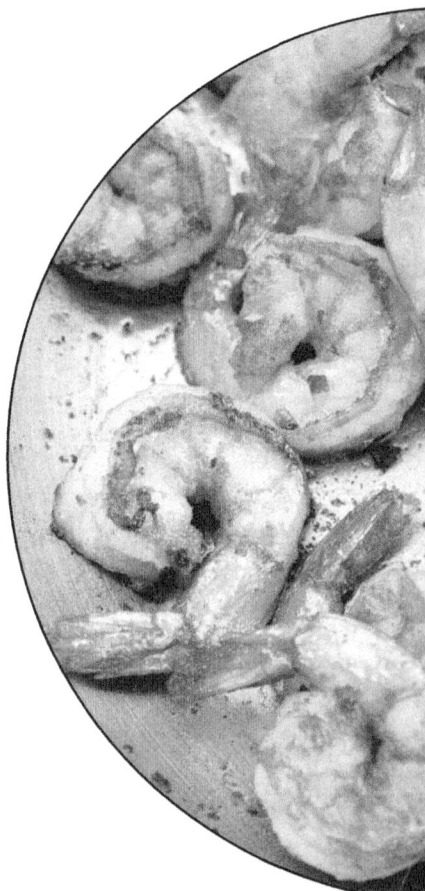

SWEET AND SPICY DOLPHIN FISH FILETS

Preparation Time: 10 minutes
Cooking Time: 25 minutes
Servings: 2

INGREDIENTS

- 2 Dolphin fish filets
- Pepper to taste
- 2 cloves of garlic, minced
- 1 thumb-size ginger, grated
- ½ lime, juiced
- 2 tablespoons honey
- 2 tablespoons sriracha
- 1 tablespoon orange juice, freshly squeezed

DIRECTIONS

1. In a heatproof dish that fits inside the saucepan, add all the ingredients. Mix well.
2. Place a large saucepan on a medium-high fire. Place a trivet inside the saucepan and fill the pan halfway with water. Cover and bring to a boil.
3. Cover the dish with foil and place on trivet.
4. Cover the pan and steam for 10 minutes. Let it rest in the pan for another 5 minutes.
5. Serve and enjoy.

STEAMED GINGER SCALLION FISH

Preparation Time: 10 minutes
Cooking Time: 30 minutes
Servings: 2

INGREDIENTS

- 3 tablespoons of soy sauce, low sodium
- 2 tablespoons of rice wine
- 1 teaspoon of minced ginger
- 1 teaspoon of garlic
- 1-pound of firm white fish

DIRECTIONS

1. In a heatproof dish that fits inside the saucepan, add all the ingredients. Mix well.
2. Place a large saucepan on a medium-high fire. Place a trivet inside the saucepan and fill the pan halfway with water. Cover and bring to a boil.
3. Cover the dish with foil and place on trivet.
4. Cover the pan and steam for 10 minutes. Let it rest in the pan for another 5 minutes.
5. Serve and enjoy.

NUTRITION

- Calories: 409.5
- Carbs: 5.5 g
- Protein: 44.9 g
- Fat: 23.1 g
- Saturated Fat: 8.3 g
- Sodium: 115 mg

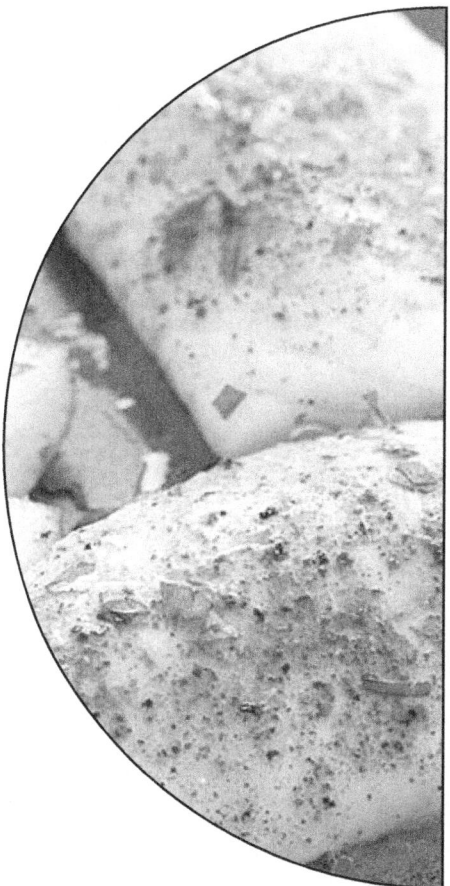

SIMPLY STEAMED ALASKAN COD

Preparation Time: 10 minutes
Cooking Time: 15 minutes
Servings: 2

INGREDIENTS

- 1-lb. of fillet wild Alaskan Cod
- 1 cup of cherry tomatoes, halved
- Salt and pepper to taste
- 1 tablespoon of balsamic vinegar
- 1 tablespoon of fresh basil chopped

DIRECTIONS

1. In a heatproof dish that fits inside the saucepan, add all the ingredients except for basil. Mix well.
2. Place a large saucepan on a medium-high fire. Place a trivet inside the saucepan and fill the pan halfway with water. Cover and bring to a boil.
3. Cover the dish with foil and place on trivet.
4. Cover the pan and steam for 10 minutes. Let it rest in the pan for another 5 minutes.
5. Serve and enjoy topped with fresh basil.

NUTRITION

- Calories: 195.2
- Carbs: 4.2 g
- Protein: 41 g
- Fat: 1.6 g
- Saturated Fat: 3 g
- Sodium: 126 mg

FISH JAMBALAYA

Preparation Time: 15 minutes
Cooking Time: 15 minutes
Servings: 2

INGREDIENTS

- 1 teaspoon of canola oil
- 1 jalapeno pepper, minced
- 1 small-sized leek, chopped
- 1/2 teaspoon of ginger garlic paste
- 1/4 teaspoon of ground cumin
- 1/4 teaspoon of ground allspice
- 1/2 teaspoon of oregano
- 1/4 teaspoon of thyme
- 1/4 teaspoon of marjoram
- 1-pound of sole fish fillets, cut into bite-sized strips
- 1 large-sized ripe tomato, pureed
- 1/2 cup of water
- 1/2 cup of clam juice
- Kosher salt, to season
- 1 bay laurel
- 5-6 black peppercorns
- 1 cup of spinach, torn into pieces

DIRECTIONS

1. Heat the oil in a Dutch oven over a moderate flame.
2. Then, sauté the pepper and leek until they have softened.
3. Now, stir in the ginger-garlic paste, cumin, allspice, oregano, thyme, and marjoram; continue stirring for 30 to 40 seconds more or until aromatic.
4. Add in the fish, tomatoes, water, clam juice, salt, bay laurel, and black peppercorns.
5. Cover and decrease the temperature to medium-low. Let it simmer for 4 to 6 minutes or until the liquid has reduced slightly.
6. Stir in the spinach and let it simmer, covered, for about 2 minutes more or until it wilts. Ladle into serving bowls and serve warm.

NUTRITION

- Calories: 232
- Total Fat: 6.7 g
- Carbs: 3.6 g
- Protein: 38.1 g

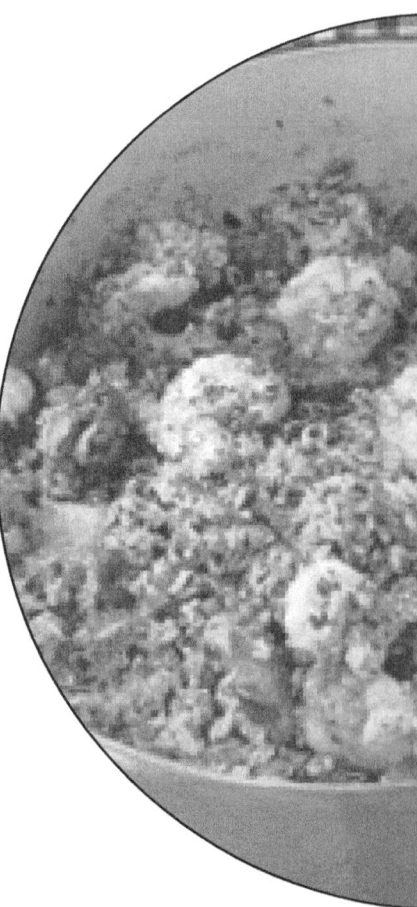

GREEK SEA BASS WITH OLIVE SAUCE

Preparation Time: 15 minutes
Cooking Time: 15 minutes
Servings: 2

INGREDIENTS

- 2 sea bass fillets
- 2 tablespoons of olive oil
- 1 garlic clove, minced
- A pinch of chili pepper
- 1 tablespoon of green olives, pitted and sliced
- 1 lemon, juiced
- Salt to taste

DIRECTIONS

1. Preheat a grill. In a small bowl, mix the half of the olive oil, chili pepper, garlic, and salt and rub onto the sea bass fillets.
2. Grill the fish on both sides for 5-6 minutes until brown.
3. In a skillet over medium heat, warm the remaining olive oil and stir in the lemon juice, olives, and some salt; cook for 3-4 minutes. Plate the fillets and pour the lemon sauce over to serve.

NUTRITION

- Calories: 267
- Total Fat: 15.6 g
- Carbs: 1.6 g
- Protein: 24 g

DINES WITH GREEN PASTA & SUN-DRIED TOMATOES

Preparation Time: 20 minutes
Cooking Time: 15 minutes
Servings: 2

INGREDIENTS

- 2 tablespoons of olive oil
- 4 cups of noodles, spiraled zucchini
- ½ pound of whole fresh sardines, gutted and cleaned
- ½ cup of sun-dried tomatoes, drained and chopped
- 1 tablespoon of dill
- 1 garlic clove, minced
- Salt and Black Pepper, to taste

DIRECTIONS

1. Preheat the oven to 350 °F and line a baking sheet with parchment paper.
2. Arrange the sardines on the dish, drizzle with olive oil, sprinkle with salt and black pepper. Bake in the oven for 10 minutes until the skin is crispy.
3. Warm the oil in a skillet over medium heat and stir-fry the zucchini, garlic, and tomatoes for 5 minutes.
4. Adjust the seasoning.
5. Transfer the sardines to a plate and serve with the veggie pasta.

NUTRITION

- Calories: 232
- Total Fat: 6.7 g
- Carbs: 3.6 g
- Protein: 38.1 g

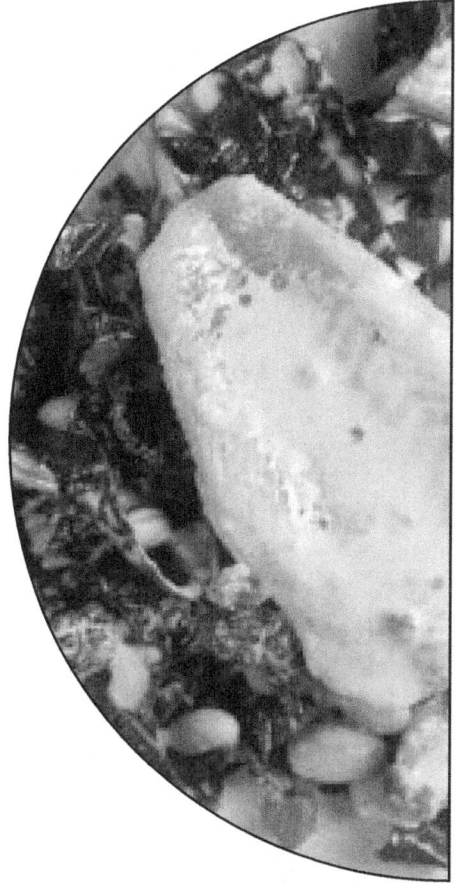

SAUCY COD WITH MUSTARD GREENS

Preparation Time: 20 minutes
Cooking Time: 15 minutes
Servings: 2

INGREDIENTS

- 1 tablespoon of olive oil
- 1 bell pepper, seeded and sliced
- 1 jalapeno pepper, seeded and sliced
- 2 stalks of green onions, sliced
- 1 stalk of green garlic, sliced
- 1/2 cup of fish broth
- 2 cod fish fillets
- 1/2 teaspoon of paprika
- Sea salt and ground black pepper, to season
- 1 cup of mustard greens, torn into bite-sized pieces

DIRECTIONS

1. Heat the olive oil in a Dutch pot over a moderate flame.
2. Now, sauté the peppers, green onions, and garlic until just tender and aromatic.
3. Add in the broth, fish fillets, paprika, salt, black pepper, and mustard greens.
4. Reduce the temperature to medium-low, cover, and let it cook for 11 to 13 minutes or until heated through.
5. Serve immediately garnished with the lemon slices if desired.

NUTRITION

- Calories: 171
- Total Fat: 7.8 g
- Carbs: 4.8 g
- Protein: 20.3 g

BAKED COD WITH PARMESAN & ALMONDS

Preparation Time: 40 minutes
Cooking Time: 30 minutes
Servings: 2

INGREDIENTS

- 2 cod fillets
- 1 cup of Brussels sprouts
- 1 tablespoon of butter, melted
- Salt and black pepper to taste
- 1 cup of crème Fraiche
- 2 tablespoons of Parmesan cheese, grated
- 2 tablespoons of shaved almonds

DIRECTIONS

1. Toss the fish fillets and Brussels sprouts in butter and season with salt and black pepper to taste.
2. Spread in a greased baking dish.
3. Mix the crème Fraiche with Parmesan cheese, pour and smear the cream on the fish.
4. Bake in the oven for 25 minutes at 400 °F until golden brown on top, take the dish out, sprinkle with the almonds and bake for another 5 minutes. Best served hot.

NUTRITION

- Calories: 560
- Total Fat: 44.7 g
- Carbs: 5.4 g
- Protein: 25.3 g

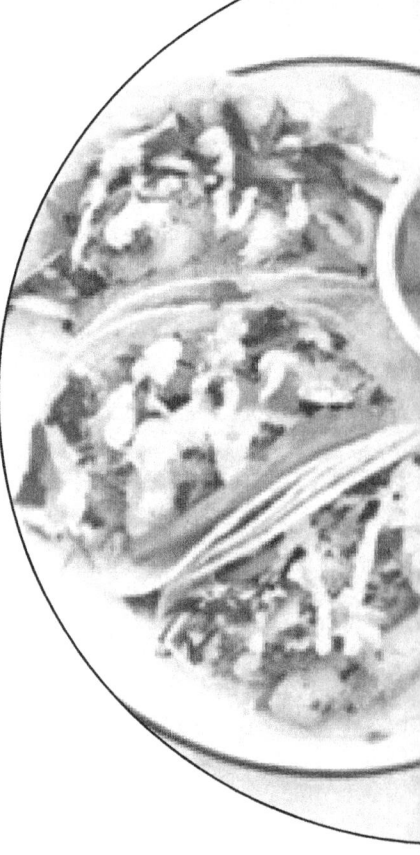

FISH TACOS WITH SLAW, LEMON AND CILANTRO

Preparation Time: 20 minutes
Cooking Time: 15 minutes
Servings: 2

INGREDIENTS

- 1 tablespoon of olive oil
- 1 teaspoon of chili powder
- 2 halibut fillets, skinless, sliced
- 2 low carb tortillas
- Slaw
- 2 tablespoons of red cabbage, shredded
- 1 tablespoon of lemon juice
- Salt to taste
- ½ tablespoon of extra-virgin olive oil
- ½ carrot, shredded
- 1 tablespoon of cilantro, chopped
- ¼ tbsp. paprika

DIRECTIONS

1. Combine the red cabbage with salt in a bowl; massage cabbage to tenderize.
2. Add the remaining slaw ingredient, toss to coat, and set aside.
3. Rub the halibut with olive oil, chili powder, and paprika.
4. Heat a grill pan over medium heat.
5. Add the halibut and cook until lightly charred and cooked through, about 3 minutes per side. Divide between the tortillas.
6. Combine all slaw ingredients in a bowl. Split the slaw among the tortillas.

NUTRITION

- Calories: 385
- Total Fat: 26 g
- Carbs: 6.5 g
- Protein: 23.8 g

FRIED OYSTERS IN THE OVEN

Preparation Time: 20 minutes
Cooking Time: 30 minutes
Servings: 2

INGREDIENTS

- 3 tablespoons of olive oil
- 1 teaspoon of garlic salt
- 1 teaspoon of freshly ground black pepper
- 1 teaspoon of red pepper flakes
- 2 cups of finely crushed pork rinds
- 24 shucked oysters

DIRECTIONS

1. Preheat the oven to 400 °F.
2. In a small bowl, mix the olive oil, garlic salt, black pepper, and red pepper flakes.
3. Put the crushed pork rinds in a separate bowl.
4. Dip each oyster first in the oil mixture to coat and then in the pork rinds, turning to coat. Arrange the coated oysters on a baking sheet in a single layer with room in between.
5. Bake in the preheated oven for 30 minutes, or until the pork rind "breading" is browned and crisp. Serve hot.

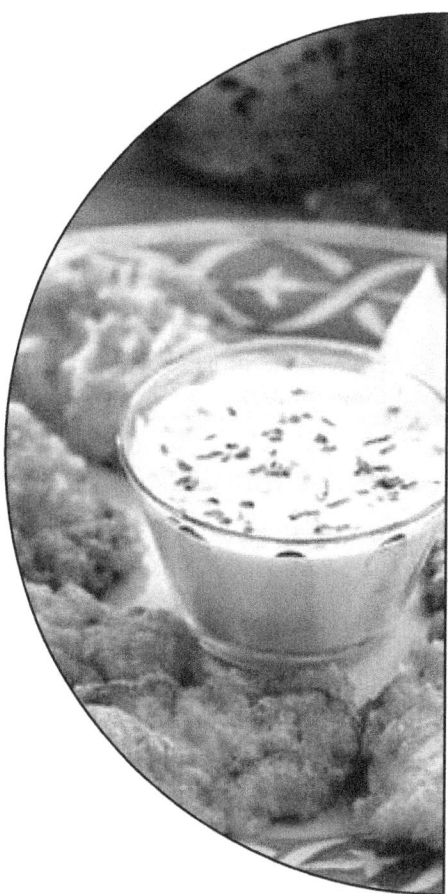

TUNA WITH GREENS AND BLUEBERRIES -ONE POT

Preparation Time: 10 minutes
Cooking Time: 5 minutes
Servings: 2

INGREDIENTS

- ¼ cup of olive oil
- 2 -4-ounces of tuna steaks
- Salt
- Freshly ground black pepper
- Juice of 1 lemon
- 4 cups of salad greens
- ¼ cup of low-carb, dairy-free ranch dressing Tessemae's
- 10 blueberries

DIRECTIONS

1. In a large skillet, heat the olive oil over medium-high heat.
2. Season the tuna steaks generously with salt and pepper, and add them to the skillet. Cook for 2 or 2 ½ minutes on each side to sear the outer edges.
3. Squeeze the lemon over the tuna in the pan and remove the fish
4. To serve, arrange the greens on 2 serving plates. Top each plate with one of the tuna steaks, 2 tablespoons of the ranch dressing, and 10 blueberries.

ROASTED OLD BAY PRAWNS

Preparation Time: 20 minutes
Cooking Time: 15 minutes
Servings: 2

INGREDIENTS

- 3/4 pound of prawns, peeled and deveined
- 1 teaspoon of Old Bay seasoning mix
- 1/2 teaspoon of paprika
- Coarse sea salt and ground black pepper, to taste
- 1 habanero pepper, deveined and minced
- 1 bell pepper, deveined and minced
- 1 cup of pound broccoli florets
- 2 teaspoons of olive oil
- 1 tablespoon of fresh chives, chopped
- 2 slices of lemon for garnish
- 2 dollops of sour cream for garnish

DIRECTIONS

1. Toss the prawns with the Old Bay seasoning mix, paprika, salt, and black pepper. Arrange them on a parchment-lined roasting pan.
2. Add the bell pepper and broccoli.
3. Drizzle the olive oil over everything and transfer the pan to a preheated oven.
4. Roast at 390 °F for 8 to 11 minutes, turning the pan halfway through the cooking time.
5. Bake until the prawns are pink and cooked through.
6. Serve with fresh chives, lemon, and sour cream.

NUTRITION
- Calories: 269
- Total Fat: 9.6 g
- Carbs: 7.2 g
- Protein: 38.2 g

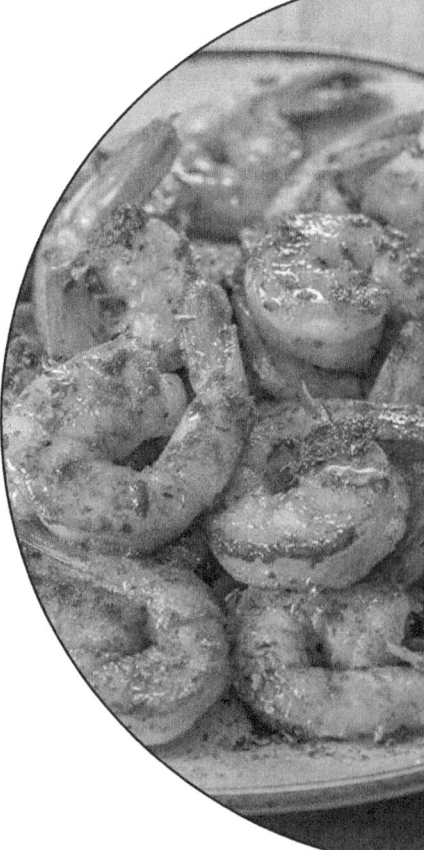

THREE-MINUTE LOBSTER TAIL

Preparation Time: 5 minutes
Cooking Time: 5 minutes
Servings: 2

INGREDIENTS

- 4 cups of bone broth, or water
- 2 lobster tails

DIRECTIONS

1. In a large pot, bring the broth to a boil.
2. While the broth is coming to a boil, use kitchen shears to cut the backside of the lobster shell from end to end.
3. Place the lobster in the boiling broth and bring it back to a boil. Cook the lobster for 3 minutes.
4. Drain and serve immediately.

NUTRITION
- Calories: 154
- Carbs: 0 g
- Fat: 2 g
- Fiber: 0 g
- Protein: 32 g

CRISPY SALMON WITH BROCCOLI & RED BELL PEPPER

Preparation Time: 30 minutes
Cooking Time: 15 minutes
Servings: 2

INGREDIENTS

- 2 salmon fillets
- Salt and black pepper to taste
- 2 tablespoons of mayonnaise
- 2 tablespoons of fennel seeds, crushed
- ½ head of broccoli, cut in florets
- 1 red bell pepper, sliced
- ¼ cup chopped carrots
- 1 tablespoon of olive oil
- 2 lemon wedges

DIRECTIONS

1. Brush the salmon with mayonnaise and season with salt and black pepper.
2. Coat with fennel seeds, place in a lined baking dish and bake for 15 minutes at 370 F.
3. Steam the broccoli and carrot for 3-4 minutes, or until tender, in a pot over medium heat. Heat the olive oil in a saucepan and sauté the red bell pepper for 5 minutes.
4. Stir in the broccoli and turn off the heat. Let the pan sit on the warm burner for 2-3 minutes.
5. Serve with baked salmon garnished with lemon wedges.

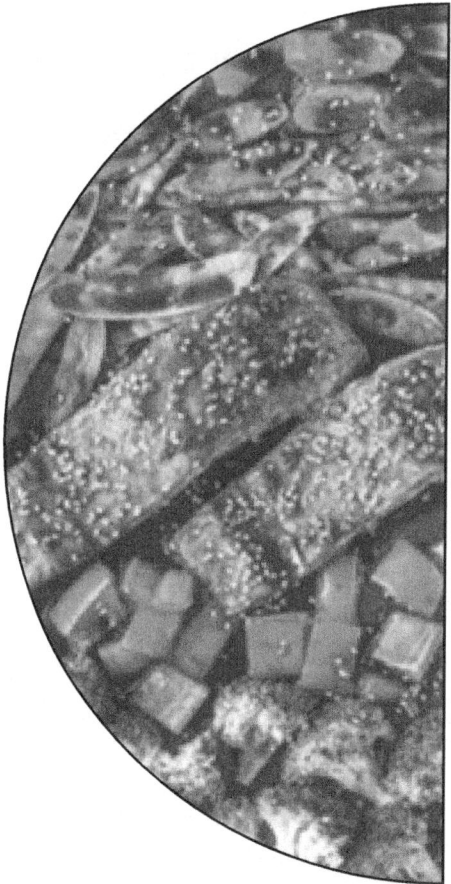

EASY BAKED HALIBUT STEAKS

Preparation Time: 20 minutes
Cooking Time: 15 minutes
Servings: 2

INGREDIENTS

- 2 tablespoons of olive oil
- 2 halibut steaks
- 1 red bell pepper, sliced
- 1 yellow onion, sliced
- 1 teaspoon of garlic, smashed
- 1/2 teaspoon of hot paprika
- Sea salt cracked black pepper, to your liking
- 1 dried thyme sprig, leaves crushed

DIRECTIONS

1. Start by preheating your oven to 390 °F.
2. Then, drizzle the olive oil over the halibut steaks.
3. Place the halibut in a baking dish that is previously greased with a nonstick spray.
4. Top with bell pepper, onion, and garlic.
5. Sprinkle with hot paprika, salt, black pepper, and dried thyme over everything.
6. Bake in the preheated oven for 13 to 15 minutes and serve immediately. Enjoy!

MEDITERRANEAN TILAPIA BAKE

Preparation Time: 20 minutes
Cooking Time: 15 minutes
Servings: 2

INGREDIENTS

- 2 tablespoons of olive oil
- 4 cups of noodles, spiraled zucchini
- ½ pound of whole fresh sardines, gutted and cleaned
- ½ cup of sun-dried tomatoes, drained and chopped
- 1 tablespoon of dill
- 1 garlic clove, minced
- Salt and Black Pepper, to taste

DIRECTIONS

1. Preheat the oven to 350 °F and line a baking sheet with parchment paper.
2. Arrange the sardines on the dish, drizzle with olive oil, sprinkle with salt and black pepper. Bake in the oven for 10 minutes until the skin is crispy.
3. Warm the oil in a skillet over medium heat and stir-fry the zucchini, garlic, and tomatoes for 5 minutes.
4. Adjust the seasoning.
5. Transfer the sardines to a plate and serve with the veggie pasta.

NUTRITION

- Calories: 232
- Total Fat: 6.7 g
- Carbs: 3.6 g
- Protein: 38.1 g

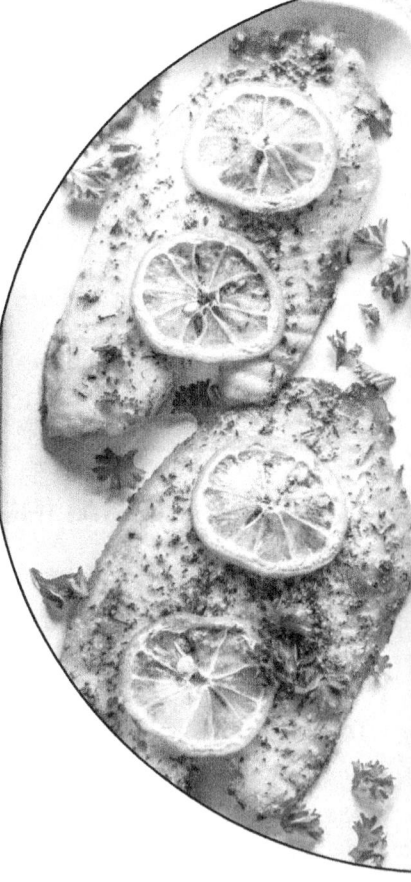

SAUCY COD WITH MUSTARD GREENS

Preparation Time: 20 minutes
Cooking Time: 15 minutes
Servings: 2

INGREDIENTS

- 1 tablespoon of olive oil
- 1 bell pepper, seeded and sliced
- 1 jalapeno pepper, seeded and sliced
- 2 stalks of green onions, sliced
- 1 stalk of green garlic, sliced
- 1/2 cup of fish broth
- 2 cod fish fillets
- 1/2 teaspoon of paprika
- Sea salt and ground black pepper, to season
- 1 cup of mustard greens, torn into bite-sized pieces

DIRECTIONS

1. Heat the olive oil in a Dutch pot over a moderate flame.
2. Now, sauté the peppers, green onions, and garlic until just tender and aromatic.
3. Add in the broth, fish fillets, paprika, salt, black pepper, and mustard greens.
4. Reduce the temperature to medium-low, cover, and let it cook for 11 to 13 minutes or until heated through.
5. Serve immediately garnished with the lemon slices if desired.

NUTRITION

- Calories: 171
- Total Fat: 7.8 g
- Carbs: 4.8 g
- Protein: 20.3 g

FRIED OYSTERS IN THE OVEN

Preparation Time: 20 minutes
Cooking Time: 30 minutes
Servings: 2

INGREDIENTS

- 3 tablespoons of olive oil
- 1 teaspoon of garlic salt
- 1 teaspoon of freshly ground black pepper
- 1 teaspoon of red pepper flakes
- 2 cups of finely crushed pork rinds
- 24 shucked oysters

DIRECTIONS

1. Preheat the oven to 400 ºF.
2. In a small bowl, mix the olive oil, garlic salt, black pepper, and red pepper flakes.
3. Put the crushed pork rinds in a separate bowl.
4. Dip each oyster first in the oil mixture to coat and then in the pork rinds, turning to coat. Arrange the coated oysters on a baking sheet in a single layer with room in between.
5. Bake in the preheated oven for 30 minutes, or until the pork rind "breading" is browned and crisp. Serve hot.

NUTRITION
- Calories: 230
- Carbs: 5 g
- Fat: 17g
- Fiber: 0 g
- Protein: 15 g

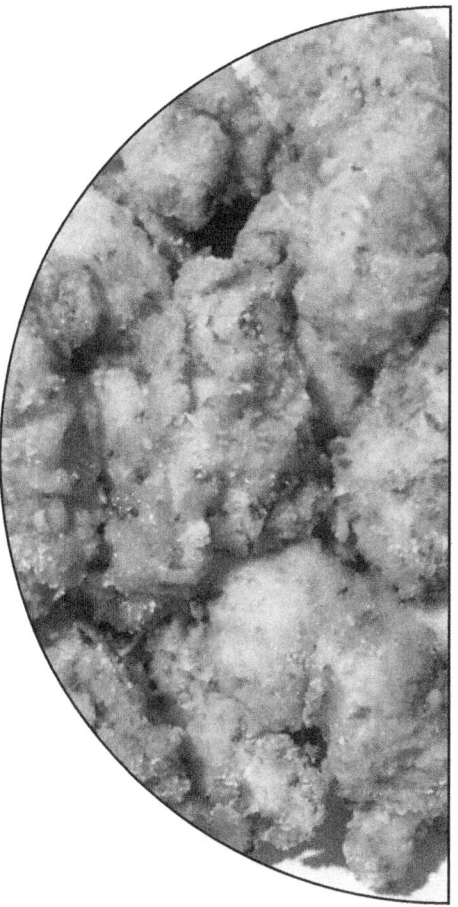

TUNA WITH GREENS AND BLUEBERRIES -ONE POT

Preparation Time: 20 minutes
Cooking Time: 15 minutes
Servings: 2

INGREDIENTS

- ¼ cup of olive oil
- 2 -4-ounces of tuna steaks
- Salt
- Freshly ground black pepper
- Juice of 1 lemon
- 4 cups of salad greens
- ¼ cup of low-carb, dairy-free ranch dressing Tessemae's
- 10 blueberries

DIRECTIONS

1. In a large skillet, heat the olive oil over medium-high heat.
2. Season the tuna steaks generously with salt and pepper, and add them to the skillet. Cook for 2 or 2 ½ minutes on each side to sear the outer edges.
3. Squeeze the lemon over the tuna in the pan and remove the fish
4. To serve, arrange the greens on 2 serving plates. Top each plate with one of the tuna steaks, 2 tablespoons of the ranch dressing, and 10 blueberries.

NUTRITION
- Calories: 549
- Carbs: 7 g
- Fat: 41 g
- Fiber: 3 g
- Protein: 38 g

MEDITERRANEAN TILAPIA BAKE

Preparation Time: 30 minutes
Cooking Time: 15 minutes
Servings: 2

INGREDIENTS

- 2 tilapia fillets
- 2 garlic cloves, minced
- 1 teaspoon of basil, chopped
- 1 cup of canned tomatoes
- ¼ tablespoon of chili powder
- 2 tablespoons of white wine
- 1 tablespoon of olive oil
- ½ red onion, chopped
- 10 black olives, pitted and halved

DIRECTIONS

1. Preheat the oven to 350 ºF. Heat the olive oil in a skillet over medium heat and cook the onion and garlic for about 3 minutes.
2. Stir in tomatoes, olives, chili powder, and white wine, and bring the mixture to a boil. Reduce the heat and simmer for 5 minutes.
3. Put the tilapia in a baking dish, pour over the sauce and bake in the oven for 10-15 minutes.
4. Serve garnished with basil.

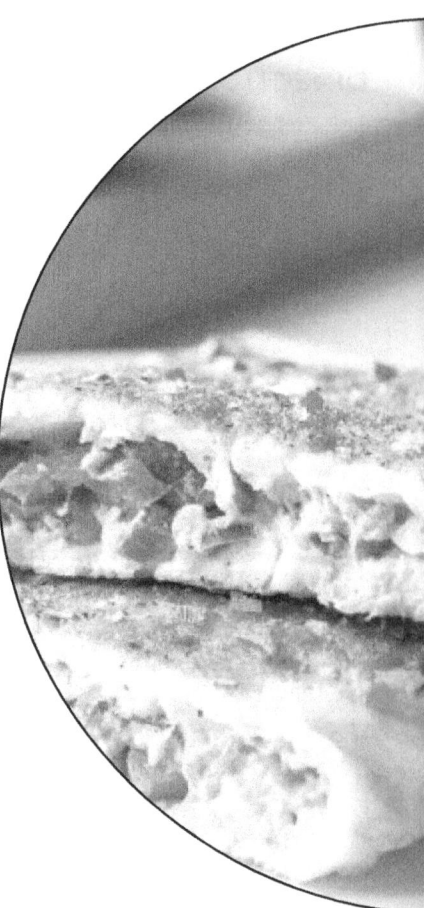

OMELET WRAPS WITH TUNA

Preparation Time: 15 minutes
Cooking Time: 15 minutes
Servings: 2

INGREDIENTS

- 1 avocado, sliced
- 1 tablespoon of chopped chives
- 1/3 cup of canned tuna, drained
- 2 spring onions, sliced
- 4 eggs, beaten
- 4 tablespoons of mascarpone cheese
- 1 tablespoon of butter
- Salt and black pepper, to taste

DIRECTIONS

1. In a small bowl, combine the chives and mascarpone cheese; set aside.
2. Melt the butter in a pan over medium heat.
3. Add the eggs to the pan and cook for about 3 minutes. Flip the omelet over and continue cooking for another 2 minutes until golden.
4. Season with salt and black pepper. Remove the omelet to a plate and spread the chive mixture over. Arrange the tuna, avocado, and onion slices.
5. Wrap the omelet and serve immediately.

BAKED TROUT AND ASPARAGUS FOIL PACKETS

Preparation Time: 20 minutes
Cooking Time: 15 minutes
Servings: 2

INGREDIENTS

- ½ pound of asparagus spears
- 1 tablespoon of garlic puree
- ½ pound of deboned trout, butterflied
- Salt and black pepper to taste
- 3 tablespoons of olive oil
- 2 sprigs of rosemary
- 2 sprigs of thyme
- 2 tablespoons of butter
- ½ medium red onion, sliced
- 2 lemon slices

DIRECTIONS

1. Preheat the oven to 400 ºF. Rub the trout with garlic puree, salt, and black pepper. Prepare two aluminum foil squares.
2. Place the fish on each square.
3. Divide the asparagus and onion between the squares, top with a pinch of salt and pepper, a sprig of rosemary and thyme, and 1 tablespoon of butter.
4. Also, lay the lemon slices on the fish. Wrap and close the fish packets securely, and place them on a baking sheet.
5. Bake in the oven for 15 minutes, and remove once ready.

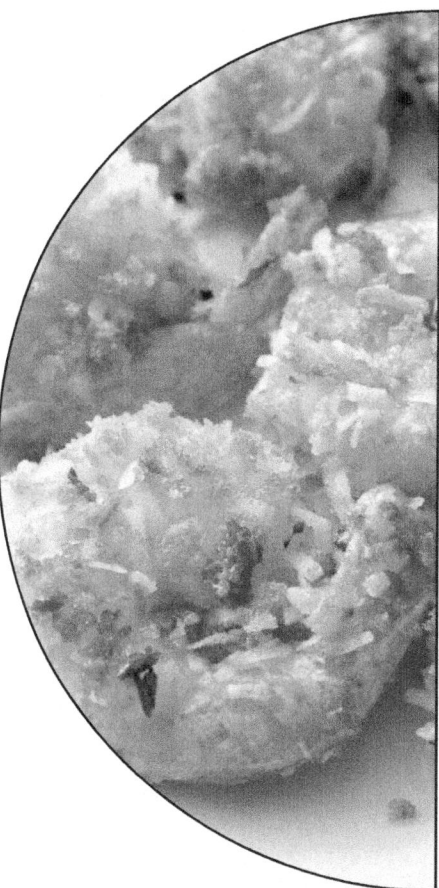

NUTRITION
- Calories: 498
- Total Fat: 39.3 g
- Carbs: 4.8 g
- Protein: 27 g

COCONUT SHRIMP

Preparation Time: 20 minutes
Cooking Time: 30 minutes
Servings: 2

INGREDIENTS

- Avocado oil spray, or another cooking oil spray
- 3 large egg whites
- 1 teaspoon of cayenne
- 1 teaspoon of garlic salt
- 1 teaspoon of freshly ground black pepper
- ½ teaspoon of Swerve granular, or another granulated alternative sweetener
- 1 cup of unsweetened shredded coconut
- 24 raw shrimp, peeled

DIRECTIONS

1. Preheat the oven to 350 ºF. Spray a large baking sheet with the avocado oil spray.
2. In a small bowl, whisk the egg whites, cayenne, garlic salt, pepper, and sweetener.
3. Put the shredded coconut in a separate bowl.
4. One at a time, dunk the shrimp first in the egg mixture and then in the coconut, turning to coat completely.
5. Arrange the coated shrimp on the prepared baking sheet in a single layer, with room in between. Once all the shrimp have been coated, spray them lightly with avocado oil spray.
6. Bake in the preheated oven for 30 minutes or until the coconut is golden brown.

NUTRITION
- Calories: 223
- Carbs: 7 g
- Fat: 17 g
- Fiber: 4 g
- Protein: 13 g

BACON-WRAPPED SCALLOP CUPS -ONE POT

Preparation Time: 10 minutes
Cooking Time: 25 minutes
Servings: 2

INGREDIENTS

- 12 large sea scallops
- 6 strips of bacon, halved to make 12 short strips
- 24 garlic cloves, peeled but left whole
- 5 tablespoons of Lemon-Garlic Dressing

DIRECTIONS

1. Preheat the oven to 400 °F.
2. Wrap each scallop with 1 piece of bacon. Use a toothpick to secure the bacon to the scallop. Arrange the wrapped scallops on a baking sheet.
3. Place 2 garlic cloves on top of each scallop, then top with a spoonful of the dressing. Bake for 25 minutes, or until the bacon is browned and crisp.

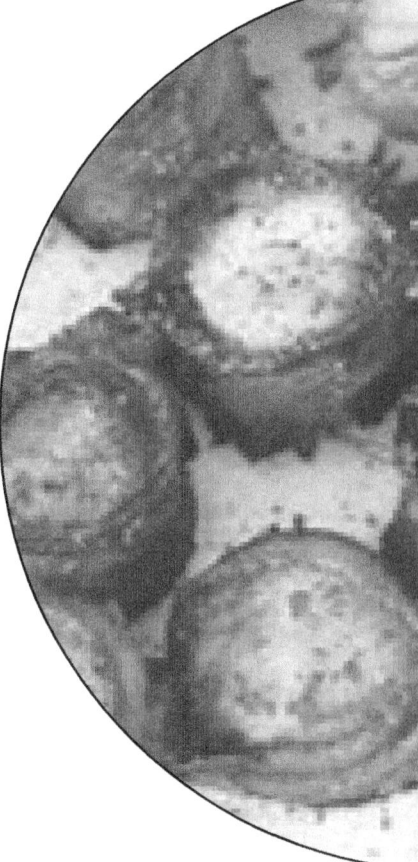

SEA BASS WITH VEGETABLES AND DILL SAUCE

Preparation Time: 25 minutes
Cooking Time: 15 minutes
Servings: 2

INGREDIENTS

- 1 tablespoon of olive oil
- 1 cup of red onions, sliced
- 2 bell peppers, deveined and sliced
- Sea salt and cayenne pepper, to taste
- 1 teaspoon of paprika
- 1-pound of sea bass fillets

Dill Sauce:
- 1 tablespoon of mayonnaise
- 1/4 cup of Greek yogurt
- 1 tablespoon of fresh dill, chopped
- 1/2 teaspoon of garlic powder
- 1/2 fresh lemon, juiced

DIRECTIONS

1. Toss the onions, peppers, and sea bass fillets with olive oil, salt, cayenne pepper, and paprika. Line a baking pan with a piece of parchment paper.
2. Preheat your oven to 400 °F.
3. Arrange your fish and vegetables on the prepared baking pan.
4. Bake for 10 minutes; turn them over and bake for a further 10 to 12 minutes.
5. Meanwhile, make the sauce by mixing all ingredients until well combined.
6. Serve the fish and vegetables with the dill sauce on the side.

GRILLED TUNA STEAKS WITH SHIRATAKI PAD THAI

Preparation Time: 30 minutes
Cooking Time: 15 minutes
Servings: 2

INGREDIENTS

- ½ pack of 7-oz. of shirataki noodles
- 2 cups of water
- 1 red bell pepper, seeded and sliced
- 2 tablespoons of soy sauce, sugar-free
- 1 tablespoon of ginger-garlic paste
- 1 teaspoon of chili powder
- 1 tablespoon of water
- 2 tuna steaks
- Salt and black pepper to taste
- 1 tablespoon of olive oil
- 1 tablespoon of parsley, chopped

DIRECTIONS

1. In a colander, rinse the shirataki noodles with running cold water.
2. Bring a pot of salted water to a boil; blanch the noodles for 2 minutes.
3. Drain and set aside. Preheat a grill on medium-high.
4. Season the tuna with salt and black pepper, brush with olive oil, and grill covered.
5. Cook for 3 minutes on each side.
6. In a bowl, whisk together soy sauce, ginger-garlic paste, olive oil, chili powder, and water.
7. Add the bell pepper and dry noodles, and toss to coat.
8. Assemble the noodles and tuna on a serving plate and garnish with parsley.

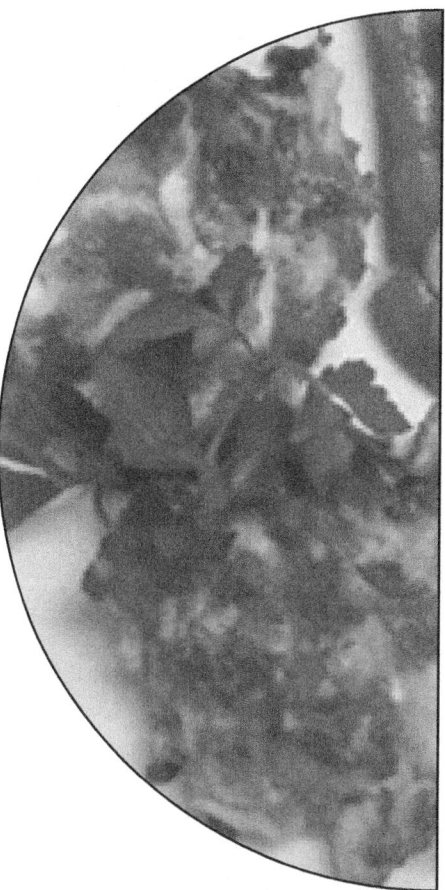

COUNTRY CLUB CRAB CAKES

Preparation Time: 30 minutes
Cooking Time: 10 minutes
Servings: 2

INGREDIENTS

- 2 -6-ounces cans of crabmeat, or 12 ounces of cooked crabmeat
- 2 large eggs
- 2 tablespoons of chopped fresh dill
- 1 teaspoon of garlic salt
- ¼ cup of olive oil

DIRECTIONS

1. In a medium bowl, combine the crabmeat, eggs, dill, and garlic salt. Form the mixture into four patties.
2. In a medium skillet, heat the olive oil over medium heat. Cook the crab cakes for 3 to 4 minutes on each side or until golden brown.

COCONUT FRIED SHRIMP WITH CILANTRO SAUCE

Preparation Time: 15 minutes
Cooking Time: 15 minutes
Servings: 2

INGREDIENTS

- 2 tablespoon of grated Pecorino cheese
- 1 egg, beaten in a bowl
- ¼ teaspoon of curry powder
- ½ pound of shrimp, shelled
- 3 tablespoon of coconut oil
- Salt to taste

Sauce
- 2 tablespoon of ghee
- 2 tablespoon of cilantro leaves, chopped
- ½ onion, diced
- ½ cup of coconut cream
- ½ ounce of Paneer cheese, grated

DIRECTIONS

1. Combine the coconut flour, Pecorino cheese, curry powder, and salt in a bowl.
2. Melt the coconut oil in a skillet over medium heat.
3. Dip the shrimp in the egg first, and then coat with the dry mixture.
4. Fry until golden and crispy, about 5 minutes. In another skillet, melt the ghee.
5. Add the onion and cook for 3 minutes. Add curry and cilantro and cook for 30 seconds.
6. Stir in the coconut cream and Paneer cheese and cook until thickened.
7. Add the shrimp and coat well. Serve warm.

NUTRITION
- Calories: 741
- Carbs: 4.3 g
- Fat: 64 g
- Protein: 34.4 g

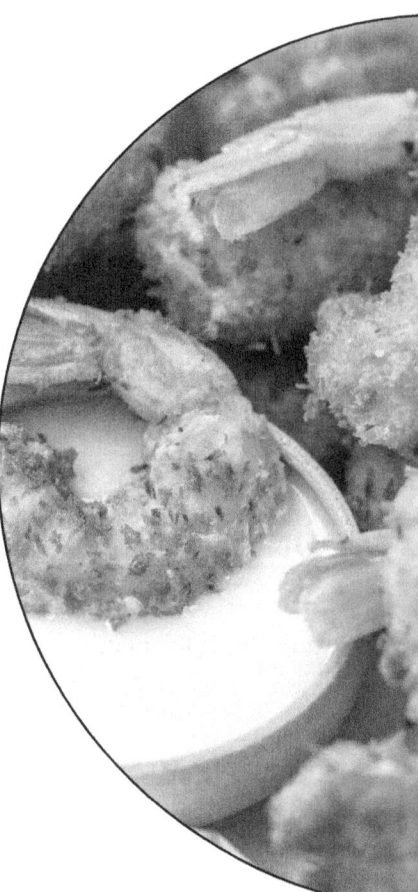

SHRIMP STIR-FRY

Preparation Time: 10 minutes
Cooking Time: 20 minutes
Servings: 2

INGREDIENTS

- ¼ cup of avocado oil
- ¼ cup of coconut aminos
- 2 cups of chopped broccoli
- 1 onion, diced
- 1 red bell pepper, chopped
- 24 cooked and peeled shrimp
- 12-ounce of cauliflower
- Chili sauce, for serving (Optional)

DIRECTIONS

1. Combine the shrimp, Cauliflower, onion, pepper, broccoli, coconut aminos, and avocado oil in a large skillet. Cook, occasionally stirring, until all the flavors are combined, about 20 minutes
2. Drizzle the chili sauce over the top and serve hot.

NUTRITION
- Calories: 231
- Carbs: 12 g
- Fat: 15 g
- Fiber: 5 g
- Protein: 12 g

BAKED SALMON WITH LEMON AND MUSH

Preparation Time: 10 minutes
Cooking Time: 30 minutes
Servings: 2

INGREDIENTS

- 2 -6-ounces of kin-on salmon fillets
- 1 onion, diced
- 8 ounces of mushrooms, sliced
- ¼ cup of olive oil
- 1 teaspoon of salt
- 1 teaspoon of freshly ground black pepper
- 4 lemon slices

DIRECTIONS

1. Preheat the oven to 400 ºF.
2. Tear off 2 large squares of aluminum foil. Place a salmon fillet on each piece of foil and arrange the onion and mushrooms over and around the fish, dividing evenly.
3. Pour the olive oil over the fish, then season with salt and pepper. Top each piece of fish with 2 lemon slices.
4. Wrap the foil up around the salmon and vegetables, leaving room inside the packet for heat to circulate, and bake for 30 minutes, or until the fish flakes easily with a fork. Serve hot.

NUTRITION

- Calories: 576
- Carbs: 8 g
- Fat: 44 g
- Fiber: 3 g
- Protein: 37 g

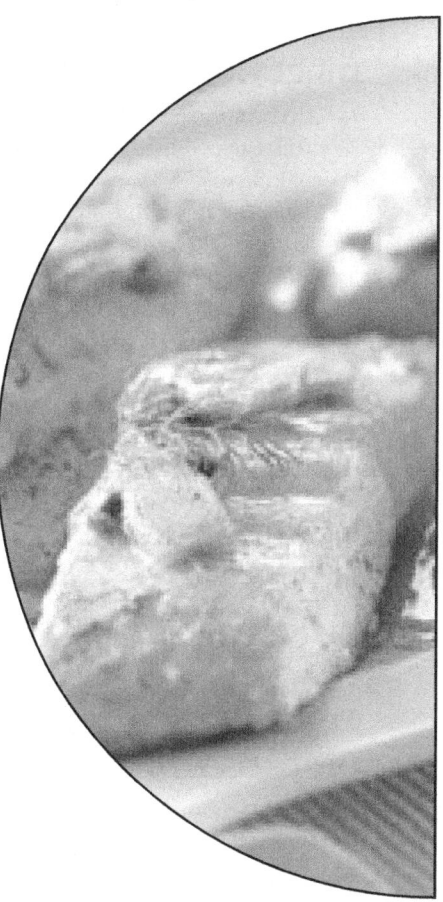

PAN-FRIED SOFT SHELL CRAB

Preparation Time: 5 minutes
Cooking Time: 10 minutes
Servings: 2

INGREDIENTS

- ½ cup of olive oil
- ½ cup of almond flour
- 1 teaspoon of paprika
- 1 teaspoon of garlic salt
- 1 teaspoon of freshly ground black pepper
- 2 soft-shell crabs

DIRECTIONS

1. Fill the bottom of a heavy skillet with the oil and heat over low heat.
2. While the oil is heating, mix the almond flour, paprika, garlic salt, and pepper in a medium bowl.
3. Dredge each crab in the flour mixture, coating both sides and shaking off any excess. Put the crabs into the hot oil in the skillet and cook for about 5 minutes per side or until golden brown.
4. Serve hot.

NUTRITION

- Calories: 489
- Carbs: 6 g
- Fat: 33 g
- Fiber: 2 g
- Protein: 42 g

CHILI COD WITH CHIVE SAUCE

Preparation Time: 20 minutes
Cooking Time: 15 minutes
Servings: 2

INGREDIENTS

- 1 teaspoon of chili powder
- 2 cod fillets
- Salt and black pepper to taste
- 1 tablespoon of olive oil
- 1 garlic clove, minced
- 1/3 cup of lemon juice
- 2 tablespoons of vegetable stock
- 2 tablespoons of chives, chopped

DIRECTIONS

1. Preheat oven to 400 °F and grease a baking dish with cooking spray.
2. Rub the cod fillets with chili powder, salt, and black pepper and lay them in the baking dish.
3. Bake for 10-15 minutes until fish fillets are easily removed with a fork.
4. In a skillet over low heat, warm the olive oil and sauté the garlic for 3 minutes.
5. Add the lemon juice, vegetable stock, and chives.
6. Season with salt, black pepper, and cook for 3 minutes until the stock slightly reduces.
7. Divide fish into 2 plates, top with sauce, and serve.

NUTRITION

- Calories: 448
- Carbs: 6.3 g
- Fat: 35.3 g
- Protein: 42 g

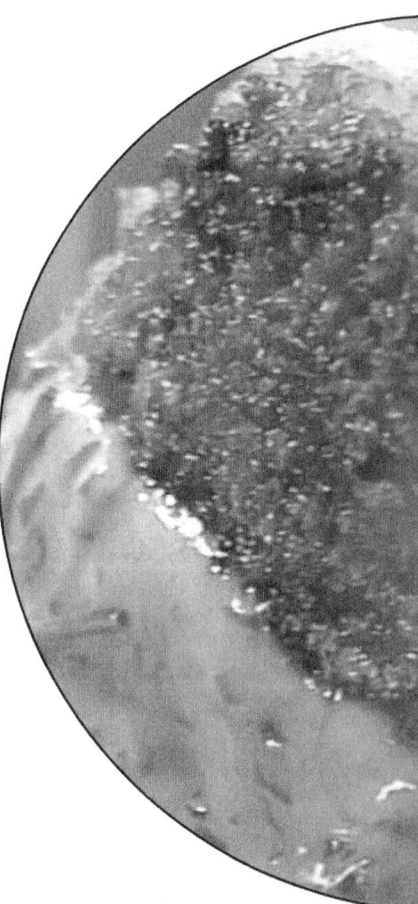

PAN-SEARED SCALLOPS WITH SAUSAGE & MOZZARELLA

Preparation Time: 15 minutes
Cooking Time: 15 minutes
Servings: 2 minutes

INGREDIENTS

- 2 tablespoon of butter
- 12 fresh scallops, rinsed and pat dry
- 8 ounces of sausage, chopped
- 1 red bell pepper, seeds removed, sliced
- 1 red onion, finely chopped
- 1 cup of Grana Padano cheese, grated
- Salt and black pepper to taste

DIRECTIONS

1. Melt half of the butter in a skillet over medium heat, and cook the onion and bell pepper for 5 minutes until tender.
2. Add the sausage and stir-fry for another 5 minutes.
3. Remove and set aside. Pat dry the scallops with paper towels, and season with salt and pepper.
4. Add the remaining butter to the skillet and sear the scallops for 2 minutes on each side to have a golden brown color.
5. Add the sausage mixture back, and warm through.
6. Transfer to serving platter and top with Grana Padano cheese.

NUTRITION

- Calories: 834
- Carbs: 9.5 g
- Fat: 62 g
- Protein: 56 g

SPANISH SHRIMP WITH A HINT OF GARLIC

Preparation Time: 5 minutes
Cooking Time: 8 minutes
Servings: 2

INGREDIENTS

- 1 pound of large shrimp, peeled and deveined
- 2 tablespoons of freshly chopped parsley
- 2 teaspoons of minced garlic
- 1/4 teaspoon of salt
- 1/8 teaspoon of ground black pepper
- ¼ teaspoon of red chili flakes
- 1 teaspoon of sweet Spanish paprika
- 11/2 tablespoon of fresh lemon juice
- 1/3 cup of olive oil
- 2 tablespoons of dry sherry

DIRECTIONS

1. Preheat a large skillet pan with oil over medium-high heat and add in garlic and red chili flakes.
2. Cook for 2 to 3 minutes until fragrant and garlic is softened, then add shrimps and season with salt, black pepper, chili flakes, and paprika.
3. Cook for additional 2 minutes or until shrimps start turning pink.
4. Stir in wine and lemon juice and continue with additional cooking for 2 to 3 more minutes or until shrimps are cooked and cooking liquid is slightly reduced.
5. Garnish shrimps with freshly chopped parsley and remove the pan from heat.
6. Serve immediately when still warm.

NUTRITION
- Calories: 834
- Carbs: 9.5 g
- Fat: 62 g
- Protein: 56 g

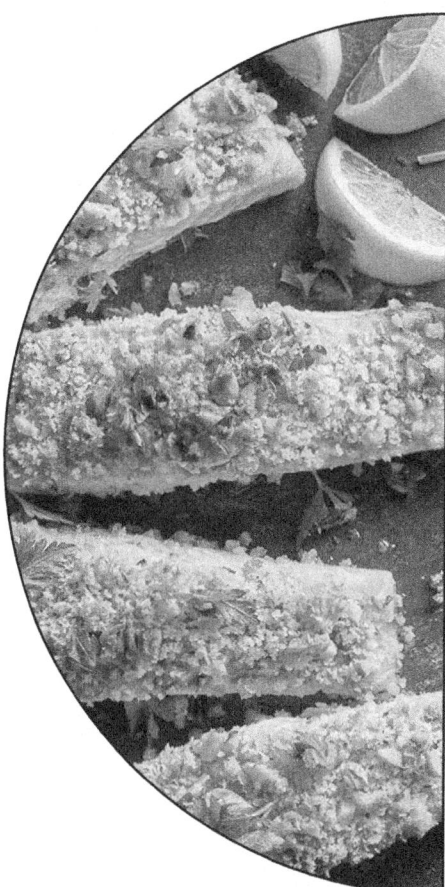

CRUSTED SALMON WITH WALNUTS AND ROSEMARY

Preparation Time: 5 minutes
Cooking Time: 12 minutes
Servings: 2

INGREDIENTS

- 1 pound of skinless salmon fillet
- 1/2 teaspoon of minced garlic
- 1 teaspoon of chopped fresh rosemary
- ½ teaspoon of salt
- ¼ teaspoon of crushed red pepper
- ½ teaspoon of honey
- ¼ teaspoon of lemon zest
- 1 teaspoon of lemon juice
- 1 teaspoon of olive oil and more as needed
- 2 teaspoons of Dijon mustard
- 3 tablespoons of panko breadcrumbs
- 3 tablespoons of finely chopped walnuts

DIRECTIONS

1. Preheat oven to 425 °F.
2. Take a rimmed baking sheet, line it with parchment paper, and place the skinless salmon fillet on it.
3. Combine the minced garlic, chopped rosemary, salt, crushed red pepper, honey, lemon zest and juice, olive oil, mustard, and finely chopped walnuts.
4. Rub the mixture on fillet and then sprinkle with panko breadcrumbs.
5. Spray fish with olive oil baking spray and place the baking sheet into the oven.
6. Bake for 8 to 12 minutes or until fish is golden brown and cooked.
7. Serve immediately while still warm.

NUTRITION
- Calories: 334
- Carbs: 9.5 g
- Fat: 62 g
- Protein: 56 g

MEDITERRANEAN SALMON WITH FENNEL AND SUN-DRIED TOMATO COUSCOUS SALAD

Preparation Time: 10 minutes
Cooking Time: 25 minutes
Servings: 2

INGREDIENTS

- 11/4 pounds of salmon fillets, skinned
- 1/4 teaspoon of salt
- 1/4 teaspoon of ground black pepper
- 4 tablespoons of sun-dried tomato pesto, divided
- 2 medium fennel bulbs, cut into 1/2-inch wedges
- 1 cup of couscous
- 3 scallions, thinly sliced
- 1/4 cup of sliced green olives
- 1 teaspoon of minced garlic
- 1 tablespoon of olive oil, divided
- 1 lemon
- 1 tablespoon of toasted pine nuts
- ½ cups of chicken broth

DIRECTIONS

1. Zest the lemon, set aside, and then cut into 8 slices.
2. Cut the salmon into four portions, season with salt and black pepper, then spread 1 ½ teaspoon of pesto on each fillet.
3. Preheat a large skillet pan with oil over medium-high heat, add half of the fennel, and cook for 3 minutes or until softened and nicely golden brown.
4. Transfer the cooked fennel to a plate, set aside. Into the same pan, add the remaining oil and fennel, cook for 3 minutes until nicely browned, and then transfer to a plate.
5. Add in the couscous and thinly sliced scallion to the pan and cook for 2 minutes or until lightly browned.
6. Add in the olives, garlic, nuts, lemon zest, remaining pesto, chicken broth, and stir until well combined.
7. Add the fennel and salmon, top with lemon wedges, reduce the heat to medium-low, cover the pan, cook for additional 10 to 15 minutes, or cook completely.
8. Serve while still warm.

NUTRITION

- Calories: 384
- Carbs: 9.5 g
- Fat: 62 g
- Protein: 56 g

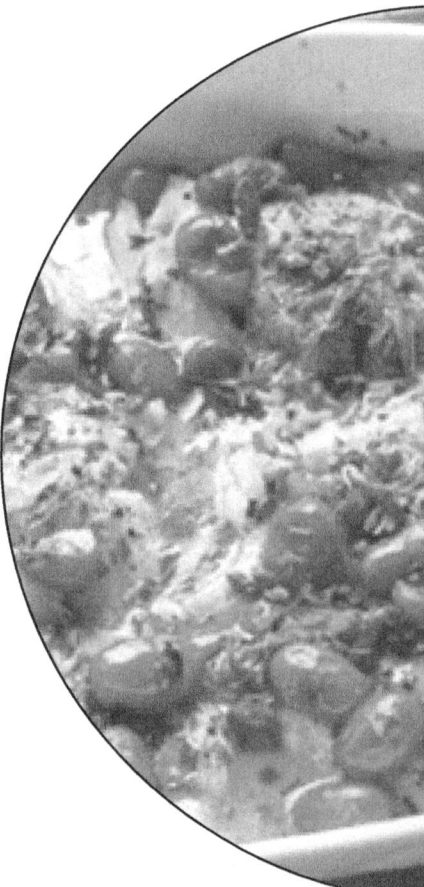

COD WITH ROASTED TOMATOES – MEDITERRANEAN STYLE

Preparation Time: 10 minutes
Cooking Time: 12 minutes
Servings: 2

INGREDIENTS

- 4 skinless cod fillets, about 4-ounce
- 3 cups of cherry tomatoes
- 2 tablespoons of sliced pitted olives
- 2 teaspoons of capers
- 2 cloves of garlic, peeled and sliced thinly
- 1/4 teaspoon of garlic powder
- ½ teaspoon of salt
- 1/4 teaspoon of ground black pepper
- 1/4 teaspoon of paprika
- 2 teaspoons of fresh oregano
- 1 teaspoon of fresh thyme
- 1 tablespoon of olive oil and more as needed Fresh oregano leaves

DIRECTIONS

1. Preheat oven to 450 º F.
2. In a bowl, mix the garlic powder, salt, black pepper, paprika, oregano, and thyme and rub half of this mixture over both sides of cod fillets.
3. Take a 15x10x1 inch baking pan, line with aluminum foil, grease well with olive oil, and place seasoned cod fillets on it.
4. Assemble tomatoes and garlic on the other side of the pan.
5. Add oil into the remaining oregano mixture, drizzle over tomatoes and mix until well coated.
6. Place the baking pan into the oven and bake for 8 to 12 minutes or until fish is cooked, stirring tomatoes halfway through the cooking process.
7. When baked, remove the baking pan from the oven, stir in olives and capers into cooked tomatoes and garlic.
8. Garnish with oregano leaves and serve while still warm.

NUTRITION

- Calories: 534
- Carbs: 9.5 g
- Fat: 62 g
- Protein: 56 g

SHRIMP PICCATA WITH ZUCCHINI NOODLES

Preparation Time: 40 minutes
Cooking Time: 10 minutes
Servings: 2

INGREDIENTS

- 1 pound of shrimp, peeled and deveined
- 2 ½ pounds of zucchini, trimmed
- 2 tablespoons of chopped fresh parsley
- 2 tablespoons of capers, rinsed
- 1 tablespoon of cornstarch
- 1 teaspoon of minced garlic
- 1/2teaspoon of salt
- 2 tablespoons of unsalted butter
- 1/4 cup of lemon juice
- 1/3 cup of white wine
- 2 tablespoons of olive oil, divided
- 1 cup of chicken broth

DIRECTIONS

1. Using a vegetable peeler cut zucchini into thin strips and place in a colander, season with salt. Toss until well coated and let rest for 15 to 30 minutes to drain all juices.
2. Meanwhile, preheat a large skillet pan with oil and butter and add in garlic.
3. Cook for 30 seconds or until fragrant and slightly softened, and then add shrimps and cook for 1 more minute.
4. Combine the cornstarch and chicken broth in a small bowl or glass and add shrimps alongside capers, lemon juice, and wine.
5. Mix well and simmer for additional 5 more minutes or until shrimps are cooked and set aside.
6. Drain zucchini noodles from their water and gently squeeze to remove any excess liquid.
7. Preheat a large skillet pan with oil over medium-high heat and add in zucchini noodles, and toss until well-coated and slightly golden brown.
8. Cook for about 3 minutes and garnish with parsley.
9. Serve the zucchini with shrimps on a serving platter.

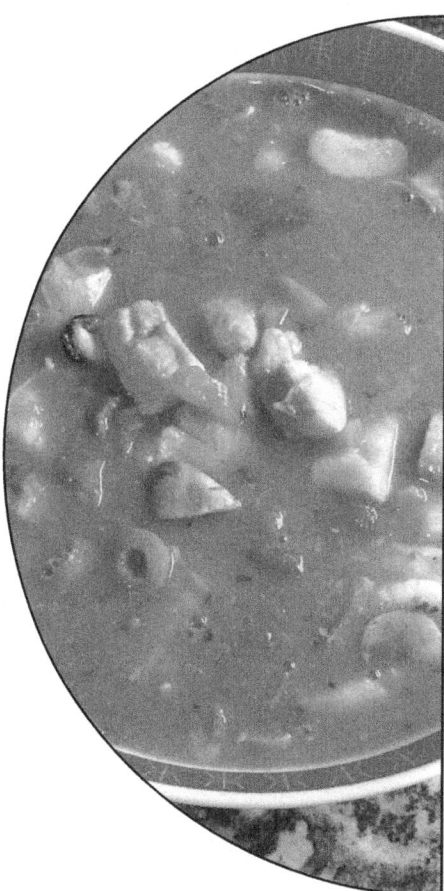

MEDITERRANEAN FISH SOUP

Preparation Time: 5 minutes
Cooking Time: 4 hours and 30 minutes
Servings: 2

INGREDIENTS

- 1 pound of cod fillets, cubed
- 1 pound of medium shrimp, peeled and deveined
- 1 medium white onion, peeled and roughly chopped
- ½ of medium green bell pepper, chopped
- 2 ½ ounces of mushrooms
- 14.5 ounces of diced tomatoes, drained
- ¼ cup of sliced black olives
- 1 teaspoon of minced garlic
- 1/8 teaspoon of ground black pepper
- 1/4 teaspoon of fennel seed, crushed
- 1 teaspoon of dried basil
- 3 pcs. bay leaves
- 1/2 cup of orange juice
- 1/2 cup of dry white wine
- 8-ounces of tomato sauce
- 28-ounces of chicken broth

DIRECTIONS

1. Turn on your 6-quart slow cooker on a low heat setting and place in chopped onion, green bell pepper, mushrooms, olives, garlic, black pepper, basil, bay leaves, crushed fennel seeds, orange juice, white wine, tomato sauce, and chicken broth. Stir well until mixed and combined.
2. Shut slow cooker with its lid, plugin and cook for 4 to 4 hours and 30 minutes or until vegetables are tender-crisp.
3. Then add shrimps and cod to vegetables and cook for an additional 20 to 30 minutes or until shrimps are pink and cooked.

CHAPTER 4.
POULTRY

EASY CHICKEN SKILLET

Preparation Time: 10 minutes
Cooking Time: 20 minutes
Servings: 2

INGREDIENTS

- 2 tablespoons of olive oil
- 4 chicken breasts, skinless and boneless
- A pinch of black pepper
- 2 tablespoons of low-fat butter
- ½ teaspoon of oregano, dried
- 3 garlic cloves, minced
- 2 cups of baby spinach
- 14 ounces of canned artichokes, no-salt-added, chopped
- ½ cup of roasted red peppers, chopped
- 1 cup of coconut cream
- ¾ cup of low-fat mozzarella, shredded
- ¼ cup of low-fat parmesan, grated

DIRECTIONS

1. Heat a pan with the oil over medium-high heat, add chicken, season with black pepper and oregano, and cook for 6 minutes on each side and transfer to a bowl.
2. Heat the same pan with the butter over medium-high heat, add garlic, spinach, artichokes, and red peppers, stir and cook for 3 minutes more.
3. Return chicken breasts, add mozzarella, parmesan, coconut cream, and toss, bring to a simmer, cook for 5 minutes more, and divide into bowls, and serve.
4. Enjoy!

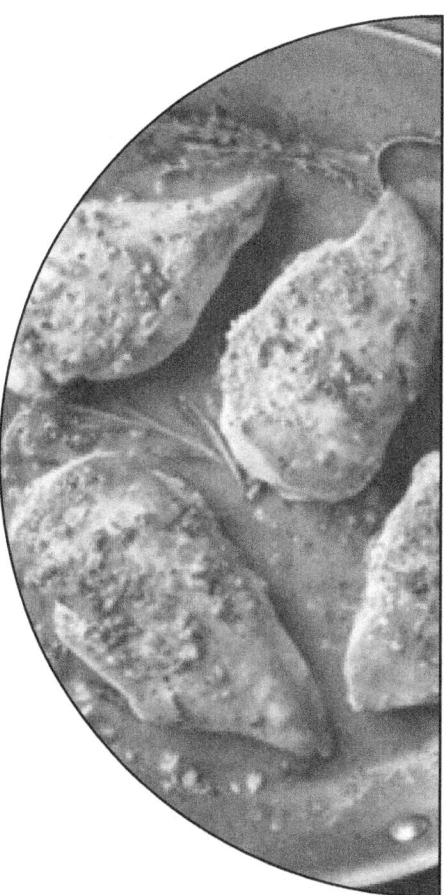

NUTRITION

- Calories: 211
- Fat: 4 g
- Fiber: 5 g
- Carbs: 14 g
- Protein: 11 g

CHICKEN AND ONION MIX

Preparation Time: 10 minutes
Cooking Time: 45 minutes
Servings: 2

INGREDIENTS

- 3 tablespoons of olive oil
- 1 yellow onion, roughly chopped
- 2 teaspoons of thyme, chopped
- 2 garlic cloves, minced
- A pinch of black pepper
- 4 chicken breasts, skinless, boneless, and cubed
- ½ teaspoon of oregano, dried
- 1 and ½ cup of low-sodium beef stock
- 1 tablespoon of parsley, chopped

DIRECTIONS

1. Heat a pan with 2 tablespoons of olive oil over medium-low heat, add the onion, black pepper, and thyme, toss and cook for 24 minutes.
2. Add garlic, cook for 1 more minute and transfer to a bowl.
3. Clean the pan, heat it with the rest of the oil over medium-high heat, add chicken, black pepper, and oregano, stir and cook for 8 minutes more.
4. Add the beef stock, add the onion mix and the parsley, toss, cook for 10 minutes, divide into bowls and serve.
5. Enjoy!

NUTRITION

- Calories: 231
- Fat: 4 g
- Fiber: 7 g
- Carbs: 14 g
- Protein: 15 g

BALSAMIC CHICKEN MIX

Preparation Time: 10 minutes
Cooking Time: 35 minutes
Servings: 2

INGREDIENTS
- 1 tablespoon of olive oil
- 1 pound of chicken thighs, bone-in, skin-on
- ½ cup of cranberries
- 2 garlic cloves, minced
- 1/3 cup of balsamic vinegar
- 2 teaspoons of thyme, chopped
- 1 teaspoon of rosemary, chopped
- Zest of 1 orange, grated

DIRECTIONS
1. Heat a pan with the oil over medium-high heat, add chicken thighs skin side down, cook for 5 minutes and transfer to a plate.
2. Heat the same pan over medium heat, add cranberries, garlic, and vinegar, thyme, rosemary, and orange zest, toss and bring to a simmer.
3. Return the chicken to the pan, cook everything for 10 minutes, introduce the pan in the oven, and bake at 325 ºF for 25 minutes.
4. Divide between plates and serve.
5. Enjoy!

NUTRITION
- Calories: 235
- Fat: 5 g
- Fiber: 6 g
- Carbs: 14 g
- Protein: 15 g

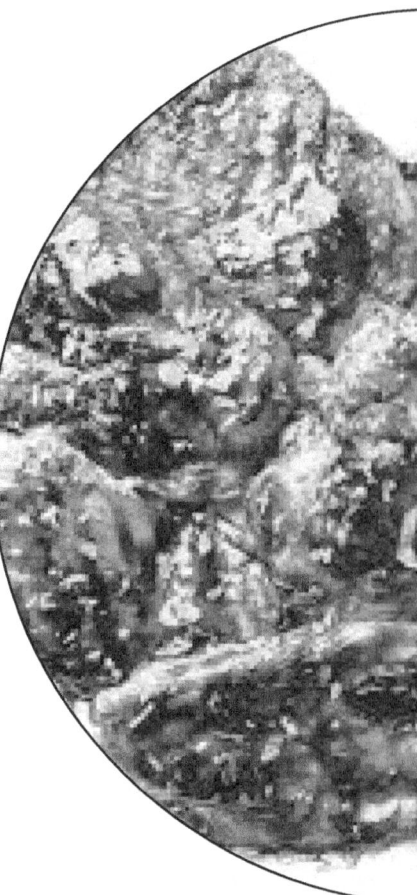

ASIAN GLAZED CHICKEN

Preparation Time: 10 minutes
Cooking Time: 30 minutes
Servings: 2

INGREDIENTS
- 8 chicken thighs, boneless and skinless
- 1/3 cup of coconut aminos
- ½ cup of balsamic vinegar
- 3 tablespoon of garlic, minced
- ¼ cup of olive oil
- A pinch of black pepper
- 1 tablespoon of green onion, chopped
- 3 tablespoons of garlic chili sauce

DIRECTIONS
1. Put the oil in a baking dish, add chicken, aminos, vinegar, garlic, black pepper, onion, and chili sauce, toss well, introduce in the oven and bake at 425 ºF for 30 minutes.
2. Divide the chicken and the sauce between plates and serve.
3. Enjoy!

NUTRITION
- Calories: 254
- Fat: 12 g
- Fiber: 6 g
- Carbs: 15 g
- Protein: 20 g

EASY GREEK CHICKEN

Preparation Time: 10 minutes
Cooking Time: 15 minutes
Servings: 2

INGREDIENTS

- 1 pound of chicken breasts, skinless and boneless
- A pinch of black pepper
- 1 tablespoon of olive oil
- 2 garlic cloves, minced
- 1 teaspoon of oregano, dried
- 1 cup of coconut milk
- 1 tablespoon of lemon juice
- 1 teaspoon of lemon zest, grated
- 1 and ½ cups of cherry tomatoes, halved
- ½ cup of calamite olives, pitted and sliced
- ¼ cup of dill, chopped
- 1 cucumber, sliced

DIRECTIONS

1. Heat a pan with the oil over medium-high heat, add chicken and cook for 4 minutes on each side.
2. Add black pepper, garlic, oregano, milk, lemon juice, lemon zest, tomatoes, olives, dill, and cucumber, toss, cook for 10 minutes more, divide between plates and serve.
3. Enjoy!

NUTRITION
- Calories: 241
- Fat: 4 g
- Fiber: 8 g
- Carbs: 15 g
- Protein: 16 g

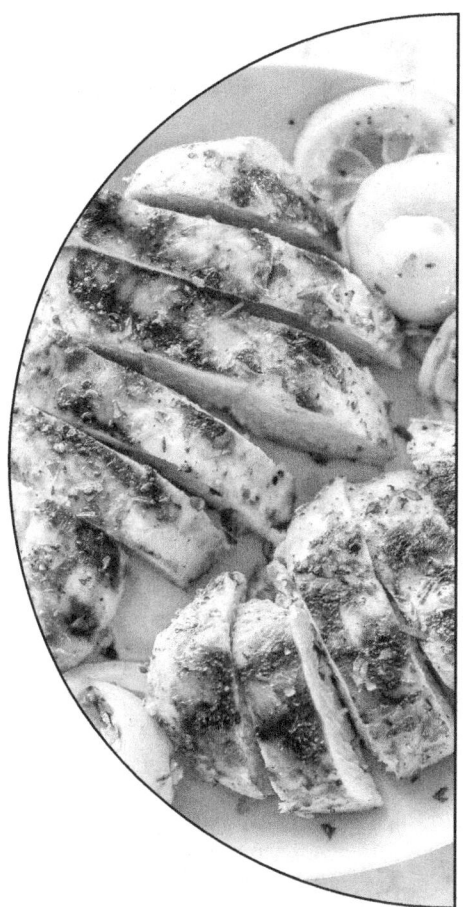

SUMMER CHICKEN MIX

Preparation Time: 10 minutes
Cooking Time: 27 minutes
Servings: 2

INGREDIENTS

- 1 tablespoon of olive oil
- 4 chicken of breasts, skinless and boneless
- A pinch of black pepper
- 1 shallot, chopped
- 2 garlic cloves, minced
- 4 peaches, sliced
- ¼ cup of balsamic vinegar
- ¼ cup of basil, chopped

DIRECTIONS

1. Heat a pan with the oil over medium-high heat, add chicken, season with black pepper, and cook for 8 minutes on each side and transfer to a plate.
2. Heat the same pan over medium-high heat, add shallot and garlic, stir and cook for 2 minutes.
3. Add the peaches, stir and cook for 5 minutes more.
4. Add the vinegar, return the chicken, also add the basil, toss, cook for 3-4 minutes more, divide everything between plates and serve.
5. Enjoy!

NUTRITION
- Calories: 241
- Fat: 4 g
- Fiber: 7 g
- Carbs: 15 g
- Protein: 15 g

CAJUN CHICKEN

Preparation Time: 10 minutes
Cooking Time: 20 minutes
Servings: 2

INGREDIENTS

- 1 tablespoon of olive oil
- 1 pound of chicken breast, skinless and boneless
- ½ teaspoon of oregano, dried
- A pinch of black pepper
- ¼ cup of low-sodium veggie stock
- 2 cups of cherry tomatoes, halved
- 4 green onions, chopped
- 1 tablespoon of Cajun seasoning
- 3 garlic cloves, minced
- ½ teaspoon of sweet paprika
- 2/3 cup of coconut cream
- 2 tablespoons of lemon juice

DIRECTIONS

1. Heat a pan with the oil over medium-high heat, add chicken and a pinch of black pepper and cook for 5 minutes on each side.
2. Add the oregano, stock, green onions, Cajun seasoning, tomatoes, garlic, paprika, cream, and lemon juice. Toss, cook for 10 minutes, divide into bowls and serve.
3. Enjoy!

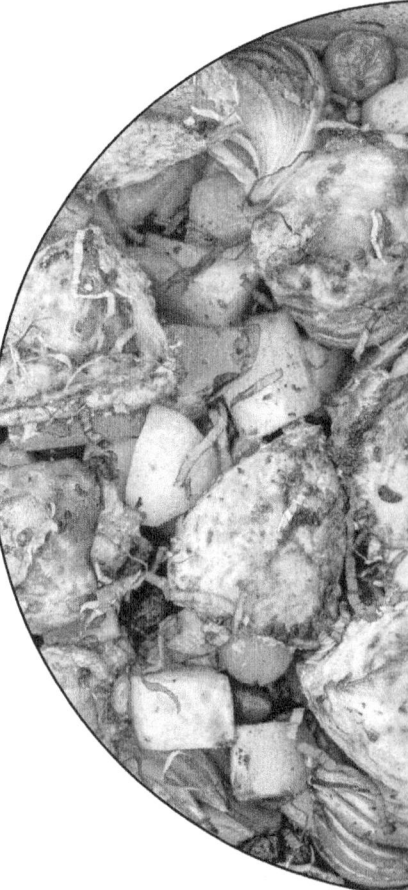

CHICKEN AND VEGGIES

Preparation Time: 10 minutes
Cooking Time: 25 minutes
Servings: 2

INGREDIENTS

- 4 chicken breasts, skinless, boneless, and cubed
- 2 tablespoons of olive oil
- ½ teaspoon of Italian seasoning
- A pinch of black pepper
- ½ cup of yellow onion, chopped
- 14 ounces of canned tomatoes, no-salt-added, drained and chopped
- 16 ounces of cauliflower florets

DIRECTIONS

1. Heat a pan with the oil over medium-high heat, add chicken, black pepper, onion, and Italian seasoning, toss and cook for 5 minutes.
2. Add the tomatoes and cauliflower, toss, cover the pan and cook over medium heat for 20 minutes.
3. Toss again, divide everything between plates, and serve.
4. Enjoy!

CHICKEN AND BROCCOLI

Preparation Time: 10 minutes
Cooking Time: 25 minutes
Servings: 2

INGREDIENTS

- 1 tablespoon of olive oil
- 4 chicken breasts, skinless and boneless
- 1 cup of red onions, chopped
- 2 garlic cloves, minced
- 1 tablespoon of oregano, chopped
- 2 cups of broccoli florets
- ½ cup of coconut cream

DIRECTIONS

1. Heat a pan with the oil over medium-high heat, add chicken breasts and cook for 5 minutes on each side.
2. Add the onions and garlic, stir and cook for 5 minutes more.
3. Add the oregano, broccoli, and cream, toss everything, cook for 10 minutes more, divide between plates, and serve.
4. Enjoy!

NUTRITION

- Calories: 287
- Fat: 10 g
- Fiber: 2 g
- Carbs: 14 g
- Protein: 19 g

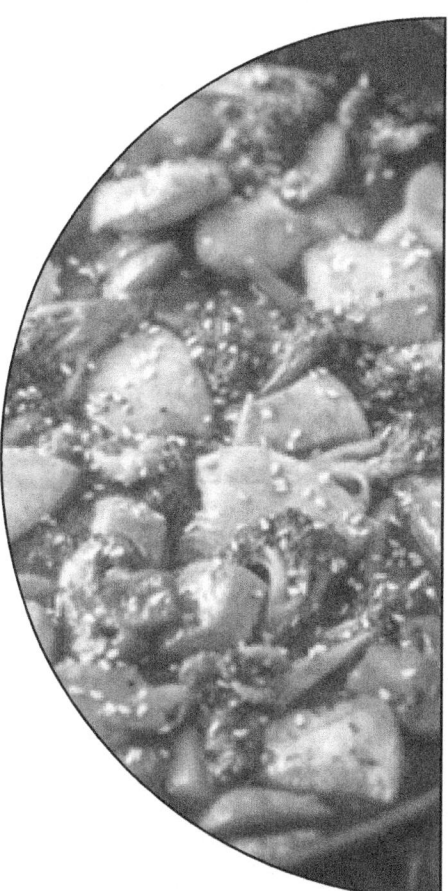

ARTICHOKE AND SPINACH CHICKEN

Preparation Time: 10 minutes
Cooking Time: 20 minutes
Servings: 2

INGREDIENTS

- 2 tablespoons of olive oil
- 10 ounces of baby spinach
- 14 ounces of artichoke hearts, chopped
- 4 chicken breasts, boneless and skinless
- 28 ounces of tomato sauce, no-salt-added
- ½ teaspoon of red pepper flakes, crushed

DIRECTIONS

1. Heat a pan with the oil over medium-high heat, add chicken and red pepper flakes and cook for 5 minutes on each side.
2. Add the spinach, artichokes, and tomato sauce, toss, cook for 10 minutes more, divide between plates and serve.
3. Enjoy!

NUTRITION

- Calories: 212
- Fat: 3 g
- Fiber: 7 g
- Carbs: 16 g
- Protein: 20 g

PUMPKIN AND BLACK BEANS CHICKEN

Preparation Time: 10 minutes
Cooking Time: 25 minutes
Servings: 2

INGREDIENTS

- 1 pound of chicken breasts, skinless and boneless
- 2 cups of water
- 1 tablespoon of olive oil
- 1 cup of coconut milk
- ½ cup of pumpkin flesh
- 15 ounces of canned black beans, no-salt-added, drained and rinsed
- 1 tablespoon of cilantro, chopped

DIRECTIONS

1. Heat a pan with the oil over medium-high heat, add the chicken and cook for 5 minutes.
2. Add the water, milk, pumpkin, and black beans, toss, cover the pan, reduce heat to medium and cook for 20 minutes.
3. Add the cilantro, toss, divide between plates and serve.
4. Enjoy!

NUTRITION

- Calories: 254
- Fat: 6 g
- Fiber: 4 g
- Carbs: 16 g
- Protein: 22 g

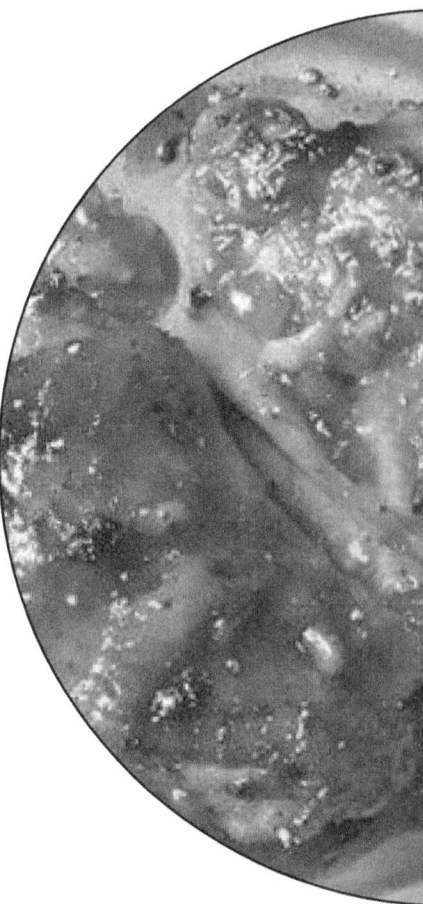

CHUTNEY CHICKEN MIX

Preparation Time: 10 minutes
Cooking Time: 10 minutes
Servings: 2

INGREDIENTS

- 4 chicken breast halves, skinless and boneless
- 2 tablespoons of lime juice
- 2 tablespoons of olive oil
- 4 tablespoons of mango chutney
- ½ teaspoon of ginger, grated
- 1 avocado, peeled, pitted, and chopped
- 8 cups of microgreens
- A pinch of black pepper

DIRECTIONS

1. In a bowl, mix chicken breasts with oil with chutney, lime juice, and ginger and toss to coat.
2. Heat your kitchen grill over medium-high heat, add chicken, cook for 5 minutes on each side, cut into thin strips, and put in a salad bowl.
3. Add the avocado, black pepper, and greens, drizzle the chutney dressing, toss to coat, and serve.
4. Enjoy!

NUTRITION

- Calories: 210
- Fat: 3 g
- Fiber: 4 g
- Carbs: 12 g
- Protein: 9 g

CHICKEN AND SWEET POTATO SOUP

Preparation Time: 10 minutes
Cooking Time: 20 minutes
Servings: 2

INGREDIENTS

- 2 chicken breasts, skinless, boneless, and cubed
- 1 yellow onion, chopped
- 2 tablespoons of olive oil
- 1 garlic clove, minced
- 4 sweet potatoes, cubed
- 2 carrots, chopped
- ½ teaspoon of ginger, grated
- ½ teaspoon of cumin, ground
- A pinch of black pepper
- 20 ounces of low-sodium veggie stock

DIRECTIONS

1. Heat a pot with the oil over medium-high heat, add onion and garlic, stir and cook for 5 minutes.
2. Add the carrots and potatoes, stir and cook for 5 minutes.
3. Add the ginger, cumin, stock, pepper, and chicken. Stir, bring to a boil, reduce heat to medium, simmer for 10 minutes, ladle into soup bowls and serve.
4. Enjoy!

NUTRITION
- Calories: 209
- Fat: 5 g
- Fiber: 5 g
- Carbs: 13 g
- Protein: 9 g

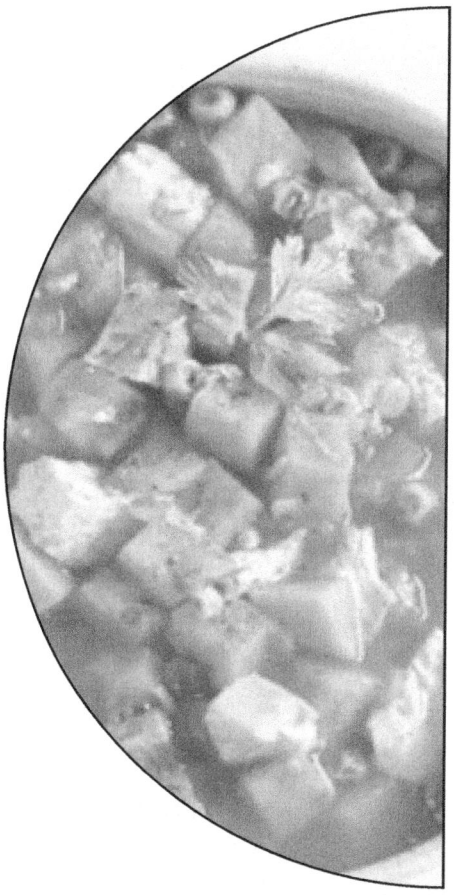

CHICKEN AND DILL SOUP

Preparation Time: 10 minutes
Cooking Time: 1 hour and 20 minutes
Servings: 2

INGREDIENTS

- 1 whole chicken
- 1 pound of carrots, sliced
- 6 cups of low-sodium veggie stock
- 1 cup of yellow onion, chopped
- A pinch of salt and black pepper
- 2 teaspoons of dill, chopped
- ½ cup of red onion, chopped

DIRECTIONS

1. Put the chicken in a pot, add water to cover, bring to a boil over medium heat, cook for 1 hour, transfer to a cutting board, discard bones, shred the meat, strain the soup, return it to the pot, heat it over medium heat and add the chicken.
2. Also, add the carrots, yellow onion, red onion, a pinch of salt, black pepper, and the dill, cook for 15 minutes, ladle into bowls and serve.
3. Enjoy!

NUTRITION
- Calories: 202
- Fat: 6 g
- Fiber: 4 g
- Carbs: 8 g
- Protein: 12 g

CILANTRO SERRANO CHICKEN SOUP

Preparation Time: 10 minutes
Cooking Time: 1 hour
Servings: 2

INGREDIENTS

- 4 chicken thighs, skin and bone-in
- 1 cup of cilantro, chopped
- 2 small Serrano peppers, chopped
- 4 and ¼ cups of low-sodium veggie stock
- 2 whole garlic cloves+ 2 garlic cloves, minced
- 2 tablespoons of olive oil
- ½ red bell pepper chopped
- ½ yellow onion, chopped
- A pinch of salt and black pepper

DIRECTIONS

1. Put the cilantro in your food processor, add Serrano peppers, 2 whole garlic cloves, and ¼ cup of stock, blend very well, and transfer to a bowl.
2. Heat a pot with the olive oil over medium-high heat, add chicken thighs, and cook for 5 minutes on each side and transfer to a bowl.
3. Return pot to medium heat, add onion, stir and cook for 5 minutes.
4. Add the bell pepper, salt, pepper, minced garlic, cilantro paste, chicken, and the rest of the stock, toss, bring to a simmer over medium heat, cook for 40 minutes, ladle into bowls and serve
5. Enjoy!

NUTRITION

- Calories: 291
- Fat: 5 g
- Fiber: 8 g
- Carbs: 10 g
- Protein: 12 g

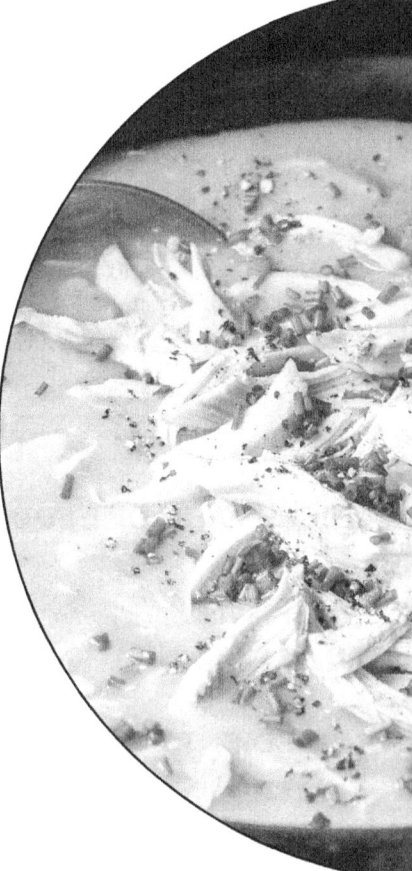

LEEK AND CHICKEN SOUP

Preparation Time: 15 minutes
Cooking Time: 1 hour and 20 minutes
Servings: 2

INGREDIENTS

- 1 lb. chicken, cut into medium pieces
- A pinch of salt and black pepper
- 3 cups of low-sodium veggie stock
- 2 leek, roughly chopped
- 1 tablespoon of olive oil
- 1/4 cup of yellow onion, chopped
- 1/8 cup of lemon juice

DIRECTIONS

1. Put the chicken in a pot, add the stock, a pinch of salt, and black pepper, stir, bring to a boil over medium heat and skim foam.
2. Add the leeks, toss and simmer for 1 hour.
3. Heat a pan with the oil over medium heat, add onion, stir and cook for 5 minutes.
4. Add this to the pot, add the lemon juice, toss, cook for 20 minutes more, ladle into bowls and serve.
5. Enjoy!

NUTRITION

- Calories: 199
- Fat: 3 g
- Fiber: 5 g
- Carbs: 6 g
- Protein: 11 g

COLLARD GREENS AND CHICKEN SOUP

Preparation Time: 10 minutes
Cooking Time: 30 minutes
Servings: 2

INGREDIENTS

- 4 cups of low-sodium chicken stock
- 1 garlic clove, minced
- 1 yellow onion, chopped
- 8 ounces of chicken breast skinless, boneless, and chopped
- 2 cups of collard greens, chopped
- A pinch of salt and black pepper
- 2 tablespoons of ginger, grated

DIRECTIONS

1. Put the stock in a pot, add garlic, chicken, and onion, stir, bring to a boil over medium heat and simmer for 20 minutes.
2. Add the collard greens, salt, pepper, and ginger, stir and cook for 10 more minutes, ladle into bowls and serve.
3. Enjoy!

NUTRITION
- Calories: 199
- Fat: 5 g
- Fiber: 5 g
- Carbs: 8 g
- Protein: 12 g

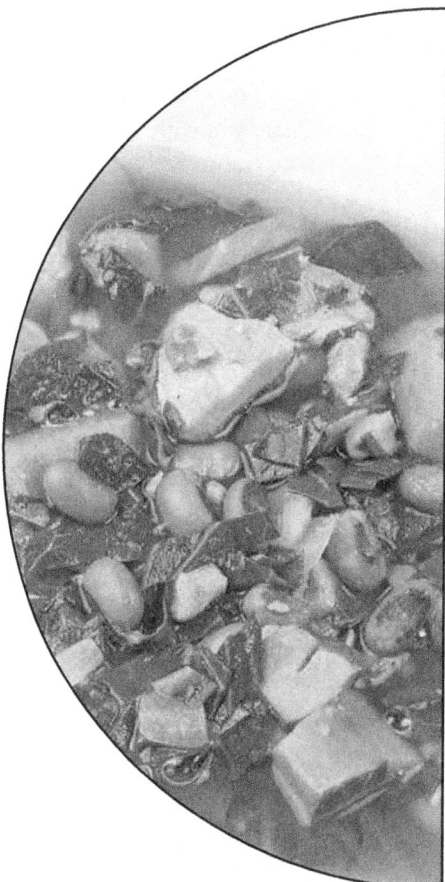

CHICKEN, SCALLIONS, AND AVOCADO SOUP

Preparation Time: 10 minutes
Cooking Time: 25 minutes
Servings: 2

INGREDIENTS

- 2 cups of chicken breast, skinless, boneless, cooked, and shredded
- 2 avocados, peeled, pitted, and chopped
- 5 cups of low-sodium veggie stock
- 1 and ½ cups scallions, chopped
- 2 garlic cloves, minced
- ½ cup of cilantro, chopped
- A pinch of salt and black pepper
- 2 teaspoons of olive oil

DIRECTIONS

1. Heat a pot with the oil over medium heat, add 1-cup of scallions and garlic, stir and cook for 5 minutes.
2. Add the stock, salt, and pepper, bring to a boil, reduce heat to low, cover and simmer for 20 minutes.
3. Divide the chicken, the rest of the scallions, and avocado in bowls, add soup, top with chopped cilantro, and serve.
4. Enjoy!

NUTRITION
- Calories: 205
- Fat: 5 g
- Fiber: 6 g
- Carbs: 14 g
- Protein: 8 g

COCONUT CHICKEN AND MUSHROOMS

Preparation Time: 10 minutes
Cooking Time: 52 minutes
Servings: 2

INGREDIENTS

- 3 tablespoons of olive oil
- 8 chicken thighs
- A pinch of salt and black pepper
- 3 garlic cloves, minced
- 8 ounces of mushrooms, halved
- 1 cup of coconut cream
- ½ teaspoon of basil, dried
- ½ teaspoon of oregano, dried
- 1 tablespoon of mustard

DIRECTIONS

1. Heat a pot with 2 tablespoons of oil over medium-high heat, add chicken, salt, and pepper, brown for 3 minutes on each side, and transfer to a plate.
2. Heat the same pot with the rest of the oil over medium heat, add mushroom and garlic, stir and cook for 6 minutes.
3. Add the salt, pepper, oregano, basil, and chicken, stir and bake in the oven at 400 °F for 30 minutes.
4. Add the cream and mustard, stir, simmer for 10 minutes more, divide everything between plates and serve.
5. Enjoy!

NUTRITION

- Calories: 269
- Fat: 5 g
- Fiber: 6 g
- Carbs: 13 g
- Protein: 12 g

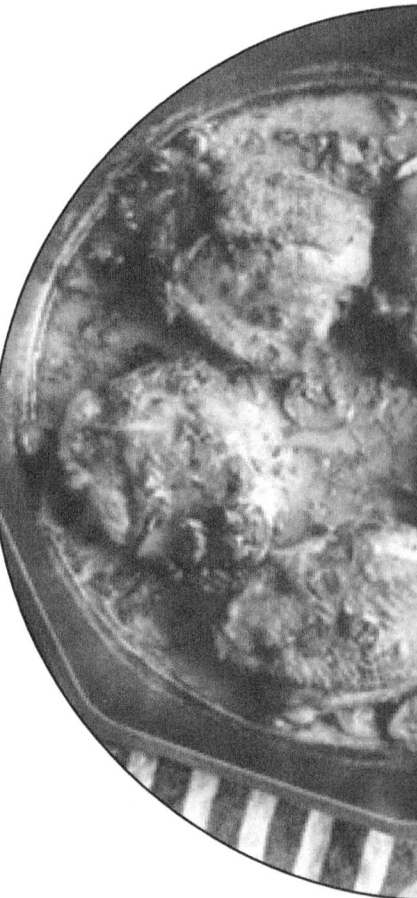

CHICKEN CHILI

Preparation Time: 10 minutes
Cooking Time: 1 hour and 10 minutes
Servings: 2

INGREDIENTS

- 1 cup of coconut flour
- 8 lemon tea bags
- A pinch of salt and black pepper
- 4 pounds of chicken breast, skinless, boneless, and cubed
- 4 ounces of olive oil
- 4 ounces of celery, chopped
- 3 garlic cloves, minced
- 2 yellow onion, chopped
- 2 red bell pepper, chopped
- 7 ounces of Poblano pepper, chopped
- 1-quart of low-sodium stock veggie stock
- 1 teaspoon of chili powder
- ¼ cup of cilantro, chopped

DIRECTIONS

1. Dredge the chicken pieces in coconut flour.
2. Heat a pot with the oil over medium-high heat, add chicken, cook for 5 minutes on each side and transfer to a bowl.
3. Heat the pot again over medium-high heat, add onion, celery, garlic, bell pepper, and Poblano pepper, stir and cook for 2 minutes.
4. Add the stock, chili powder, salt, pepper, chicken, and tea bags, stir, bring to a simmer, reduce heat to medium-low, cover and cook for 1 hour.
5. Discard tea bags, add cilantro, stir, ladle into bowls and serve.
6. Enjoy!

NUTRITION

- Calories: 205
- Fat: 8 g
- Fiber: 3 g
- Carbs: 12 g
- Protein: 6 g

CHICKEN, SPINACH AND ASPARAGUS SOUP

Preparation Time: 10 minutes
Cooking Time: 30 minutes
Servings: 2

INGREDIENTS

- 2 chicken breasts, cooked, skinless, boneless and shredded
- 1 tablespoon of olive oil
- A pinch of salt and black pepper
- 1 yellow onion, finely chopped
- 2 carrots, chopped
- 3 garlic cloves, minced
- 4 cups of spinach
- 12 asparagus spears, chopped
- 6 cups of low-sodium veggie stock
- Zest of ½ lime, grated
- 1 handful cilantro, chopped

DIRECTIONS

1. Heat a pot with the oil over medium heat, add onions, stir and cook for 5 minutes.
2. Add the carrots, garlic and asparagus, stir and cook for 5 minutes.
3. Add the spinach, salt, pepper, stock, and chicken, stir and cook for 20 minutes.
4. Add the lime zest and cilantro. Stir soup again, ladle into bowls and serve.
5. Enjoy!

NUTRITION
- Calories: 245
- Fat: 2 g
- Fiber: 3 g
- Carbs: 5 g
- Protein: 6 g

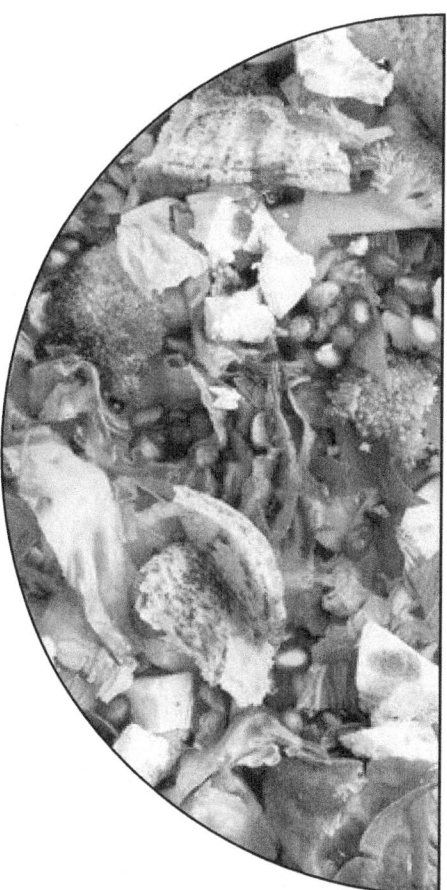

CHICKEN AND BROCCOLI SALAD

Preparation Time: 10 minutes
Cooking Time: 10 minutes
Servings: 2

INGREDIENTS

- 3 medium chicken breasts, skinless, boneless, and cut into thin strips
- 12 ounces of broccoli florets, roughly chopped
- 5 tablespoon of olive oil
- A pinch of salt and black pepper
- 2 tablespoon of vinegar
- 1 and ½ cups of peaches, pitted and sliced
- 1 tablespoon of chives, chopped
- 2 bacon slices, cooked and crumbled

DIRECTIONS

1. In a salad bowl, mix 4 tablespoon of oil with vinegar, salt, pepper, broccoli, peaches, and toss.
2. Heat a pan with the rest of the oil over medium-high heat, add chicken, season with salt and pepper, cook for 5 minutes on each side, transfer to the salad bowl, add bacon and chives, toss and serve.
3. Enjoy!

NUTRITION
- Calories: 210
- Fat: 12 g
- Fiber: 3 g
- Carbs: 10 g
- Protein: 23 g

GARLICKY ZUCCHINI-TURKEY CASSEROLE

Preparation Time: 10 minutes
Cooking Time: 40 minutes
Servings: 2

INGREDIENTS

- 1 tablespoon of oil
- 1 white onion, chopped
- 2 cloves of garlic, minced
- 1-pound cooked turkey meat, shredded
- A dash of rosemary
- 1 zucchini, chopped
- 1 carrot, peeled and chopped
- ½ cup water
- Pepper to taste

DIRECTIONS

1. Preheat oven to 400 °F.
2. Grease an oven-safe casserole dish with oil.
3. Mix the onion, garlic, turkey, pepper, salt, and rosemary in a bowl.
4. Pour into prepared casserole dish.
5. Sprinkle carrot on top, followed by zucchini, and then pour water over the mixture.
6. Cover the dish with a foil and bake for 25 minutes or until bubbly hot.
7. Remove foil, return to oven, and broil the top for 2 minutes on high.
8. Let it rest for 10 minutes.
9. Serve and enjoy.

NUTRITION

- Calories: 250
- Carbs: 5.7 g
- Protein: 32.9 g
- Fat: 10.0 g
- Saturated Fat: 2.8 g
- Sodium: 88 mg

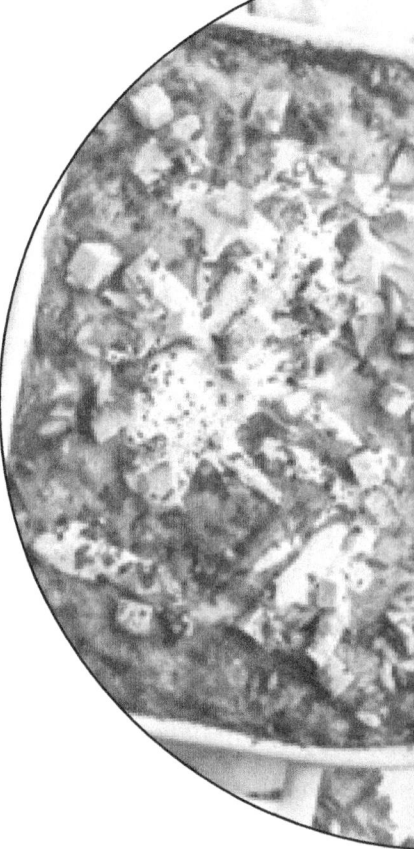

CASSEROLE A LA CHICKEN ENCHILADA

Preparation Time: 10 minutes
Cooking Time: 6 hours
Servings: 2

INGREDIENTS

- 5 pitted dates
- 3 tablespoons of olive oil
- ¼ cup of chili powder
- 1 cup of water
- 1 cup of tomato paste
- 1 teaspoon of ground cumin
- 1 teaspoon of dried oregano
- Salt and pepper to taste
- 2 pounds of chicken breasts, cut into strips
- 1 sweet potato, scrubbed and chopped

DIRECTIONS

1. In a blender or food processor, place the dates, olive oil, chili powder, water, tomato paste, cumin, and oregano. Season with salt and pepper to taste. Pulse until smooth. This will be the enchilada sauce.
2. On the Crock-Pot, place the chicken breasts and sweet potatoes on the bottom of the pot.
3. Pour over chicken the enchilada sauce.
4. Close the lid, press the low settings, and adjust the cooking time to 6 hours.
5. Serve and enjoy.

NUTRITION

- Calories: 240
- Carbs: 12.2 g
- Protein: 30.2 g
- Fat: 8.0 g
- Saturated Fat: 2.7 g
- Sodium: 204 mg

CILANTRO-COCONUT CHICKEN STEW

Preparation Time: 10 minutes
Cooking Time: 30 minutes
Servings: 2

INGREDIENTS

- 1 whole chicken, around 2-lbs
- 1 can of light coconut milk
- 1 cup of water
- ½ fresh cilantro, chopped
- 1 tablespoon of ginger
- 1 teaspoon of cumin
- 1 teaspoon of coriander
- ½ teaspoon of salt
- ½ teaspoon of curry
- 1 lemon, juice extracted

DIRECTIONS

1. Place a heavy bottomed pot on a medium-high fire.
2. Add all the ingredients except for coconut milk. Mix well.
3. Bring to a boil. Once boiling, lower the fire to a simmer and cook for 20 minutes.
4. Stir in coconut milk. Continue simmering for another 10 minutes.
5. Serve and enjoy.

NUTRITION
- Calories: 194
- Carbs: 2.3 g
- Protein: 23.8 g
- Fat: 9.9 g
- Saturated Fat: 6.7 g
- Sodium: 236 mg

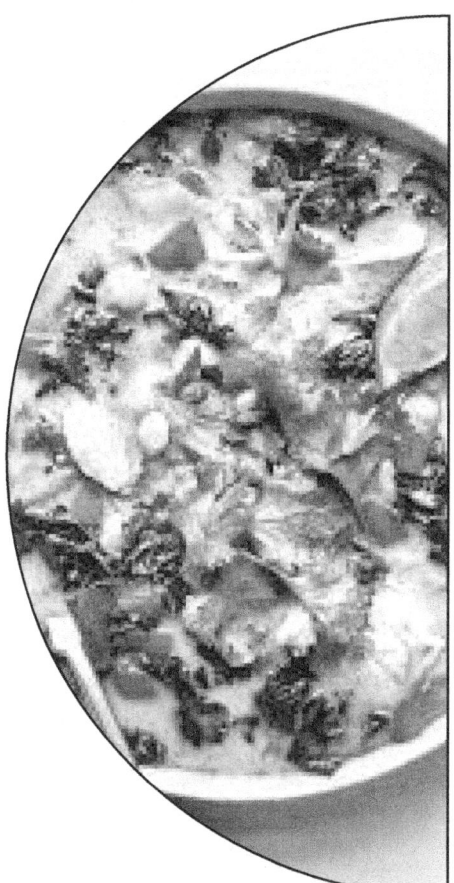

TURKEY LEGS IN THAI SAUCE

Preparation Time: 10 minutes
Cooking Time: 30 minutes
Servings: 2

INGREDIENTS

- 1 ½ pound of large turkey legs
- 1 can of light coconut milk
- 1 cup of water
- 1 ½ teaspoon of lemon juice
- ¼ cup of cilantro, chopped
- Pepper to taste

DIRECTIONS

1. Place a heavy bottomed pot on a medium-high fire.
2. Add all the ingredients except for coconut milk. Mix well.
3. Bring to a boil. Once boiling, lower the fire to a simmer and cook for 20 minutes.
4. Stir in the coconut milk. Continue simmering for another 10 minutes.
5. Serve and enjoy.

NUTRITION
- Calories: 236
- Carbs: 2.5 g
- Protein: 23.0 g
- Fat: 14.8 g
- Saturated Fat: 3.8 g
- Sodium: 90 mg

FILLING TURKEY CHILI RECIPE

Preparation Time: 10 minutes
Cooking Time: 25 minutes
Servings: 2

INGREDIENTS

- 1 tablespoon of olive oil
- 1-pound of ground turkey
- 1 onion, chopped
- 1 green bell pepper, seeded and chopped
- 3 carrots, peeled and chopped
- 2 stalks of celery, sliced thinly
- 1 cup of chopped tomatoes
- 3 Poblano chilies, chopped
- ½ cup of water
- 3 tablespoons of chili powder
- 1 ½ teaspoon of ground cumin
- Pepper to taste

DIRECTIONS

1. Place a heavy bottomed pot on medium-high fire and heat for 3 minutes.
2. Add the oil; swirl to coat bottom and sides of the pot, and heat for a minute.
3. Stir in the turkey. Brown and crumble for 8 minutes. Season generously with pepper. Discard excess fat.
4. Add all the ingredients. Mix well.
5. Bring to a boil. Once boiling, lower the fire to a simmer and cook for 10 minutes.
6. Serve and enjoy.

NUTRITION

- Calories: 175
- Carbs: 8.7 g
- Protein: 16.4 g
- Fat: 9.1 g
- Saturated Fat: 2.0 g
- Sodium: 188 mg

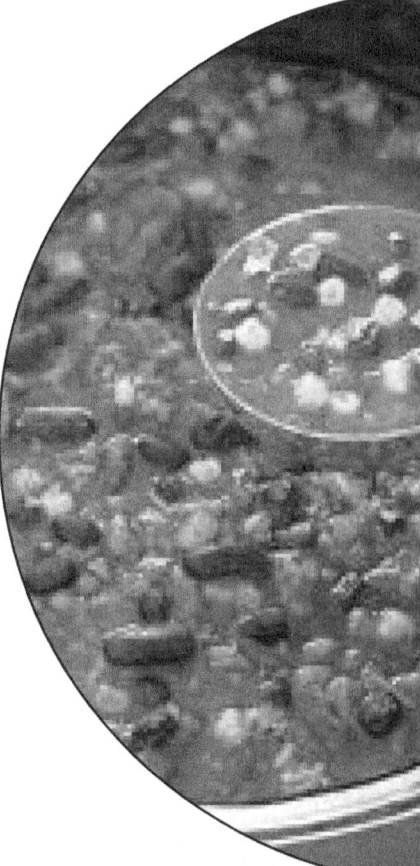

CHICKEN MEATLOAF WITH A TROPICAL TWIST

Preparation Time: 10 minutes
Cooking Time: 45 minutes
Servings: 2

INGREDIENTS

- 1/8 teaspoon of salt
- 1/8 teaspoon of pepper
- 2 eggs
- ¼ cup of parsley, chopped
- ¼ cup of coconut flakes
- ½ tablespoons of jalapeno, seeded and diced
- ½ cups of diced mango
- 1 cup of yellow bell pepper, diced
- 1-pound of ground chicken
- 1 tablespoon of oil

DIRECTIONS

1. Preheat oven to 400 °F and lightly grease a loaf pan with oil.
2. In a large bowl, mix the remaining ingredients.
3. Evenly spread in a prepared pan and cover the pan with foil.
4. Pop in the oven and bake for 30 minutes.
5. Remove foil and broil the top for 3 minutes.
6. Let it sit for 10 minutes.
7. Serve and enjoy.

NUTRITION

- Calories: 301
- Carbs: 8 g
- Protein: 25 g
- Fat: 19 g
- Saturated Fat: 4.6 g
- Sodium: 215 mg

CHICKEN-MUSHROOM CASSEROLE

Preparation Time: 10 minutes
Cooking Time: 35 minutes
Servings: 2

INGREDIENTS

- 2 tablespoon of chopped fresh parsley
- 4 slices Muenster cheese
- 1 garlic clove, minced
- 1-lb. of sliced fresh mushrooms
- 1 cup of water
- 1 18-oz. can of creamy mushroom soup, low sodium
- 1 chicken breast, sliced thinly
- ¼ teaspoon of pepper
- 2 tablespoon of all-purpose flour

DIRECTIONS

1. Place a nonstick saucepan on medium-high fire and heat for 3 minutes.
2. Add the oil and swirl the pan to coat sides and bottom with oil Heat for a minute.
3. Add the chicken and sauté until no longer pink, around 5 minutes. Season with pepper and transfer to a plate.
4. In the same pan, add flour and sauté for 3 minutes. Add garlic and sauté for a minute more.
5. Stir in mushrooms and cook for 5 minutes until water comes out of it.
6. Add the remaining ingredients, except for cheese and parsley. Mix well. Return chicken to pan.
7. Bring to a simmer, cover and cook for 10 minutes while mixing frequently.
8. Place the cheese on top and let it rest while covered for 5 minutes.
9. Serve and enjoy with a sprinkle of parsley.

NUTRITION

- Calories: 346
- Carbs: 14.7 g
- Protein: 36.4 g
- Fat: 16.3 g
- Saturated Fat: 6.8 g
- Sodium: 109 mg

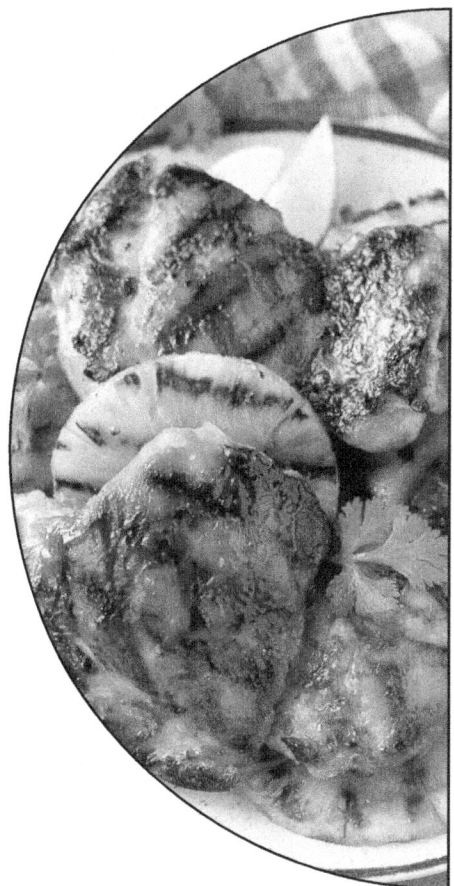

PINEAPPLE CHICKEN HAWAIIAN STYLE

Preparation Time: 10 minutes
Cooking Time: 40 minutes
Servings: 2

INGREDIENTS

- 2 tablespoon of cornstarch
- 1 small yellow bell pepper, cut into 1-inch pieces
- 1 small red bell pepper, cut into 1-inch pieces
- 1 20-oz. can of pineapple chunks, drained and ¼ cup liquid reserved
- 1 cup of honey BBQ sauce
- 2 cloves of garlic, chopped finely
- 1.5-lbs. of boneless, skinless chicken thighs
- 1 teaspoon of oil

DIRECTIONS

1. Place a heavy bottomed pot on medium-high fire and heat pot for 3 minutes.
2. Once hot, add oil and stir around to coat the pot with oil.
3. Add the chicken and cook for 4 minutes per side.
4. Meanwhile, in a bowl, mix the cornstarch with ¼ cup water and set aside
5. Add the pineapple chunks to the pot and sauté for 2 minutes.
6. Stir in reserved liquid from pineapple, BBQ sauce, and garlic. Mix well and bring to a boil.
7. Cover and lower the fire to a simmer and simmer for 8 minutes.
8. Stir in bell peppers and cornstarch slurry. Continue mixing and cooking until sauce has thickened, around 5 minutes.
9. Serve and enjoy.

NUTRITION

- Calories: 402
- Carbs: 45.9 g
- Protein: 28.7 g
- Fat: 11.6 g
- Saturated Fat: 3.0 g
- Sodium: 285 mg

HONEY SESAME CHICKEN

Preparation Time: 10 minutes
Cooking Time: 20 minutes
Servings: 2

INGREDIENTS

- 1 tablespoon of toasted sesame seeds
- 2 green onions, chopped
- 3 tablespoon of water
- 2 tablespoon of cornstarch
- ¼ teaspoon of red pepper flakes
- ½ cup of honey
- 2 teaspoon of sesame oil
- 1-inch cubes
- ¼ ketchup
- 2 tablespoon of soy sauce
- 2 garlic cloves, minced
- ½ cup of onion, diced
- 1 teaspoon of olive oil
- Pepper to taste
- 2 medium boneless, skinless chicken breasts, chopped into

DIRECTIONS

1. Place a heavy-bottomed pot on medium-high fire and heat the pot for 3 minutes.
2. Meanwhile, season chicken generously with pepper.
3. Once hot, add oil and stir around to coat the pot with oil.
4. Stir in the garlic and onion. Cook for 3 minutes.
5. Add the chicken and cook for 5 minutes.
6. Stir in the red pepper flakes, ketchup, and soy sauce. Mix well.
7. Cover, bring to a boil, lower the fire to a simmer, and simmer for 5 minutes.
8. Meanwhile, in a bowl, mix cornstarch with water and set aside
9. Stir in honey, sesame seeds and sesame oil. Pour the cornstarch slurry and continue mixing while cooking until sauce has thickened around 5 minutes.
10. Serve and enjoy with a sprinkle of green onions.

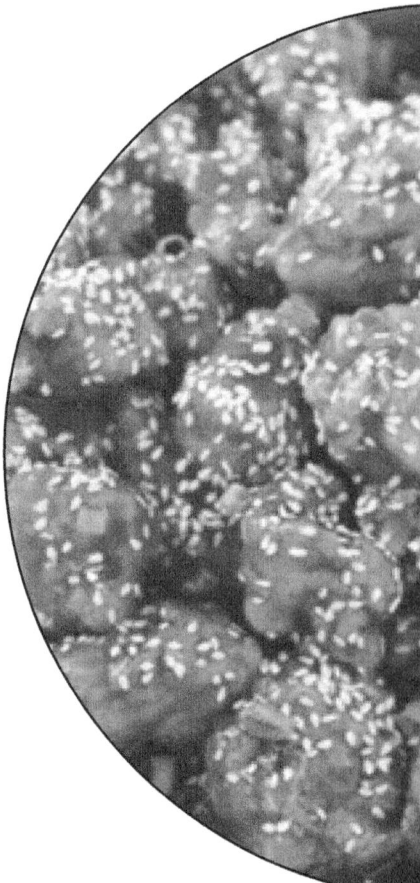

NUTRITION

- Calories: 228
- Carbs: 44.7 g
- Protein: 3.9 g
- Fat: 5.4 g
- Saturated Fat: 0.8 g
- Sodium: 304 mg

CHICKEN COOKED THE ITALIAN WAY

Preparation Time: 10 minutes
Cooking Time: 25 minutes
Servings: 2

INGREDIENTS

- ¼ cup of loosely packed fresh Italian parsley, chopped coarsely
- ½ cup of loosely packed fresh basil leaves, sliced thinly
- ¼ teaspoon of black pepper
- ½ cup of pitted green olives
- 2 cups of cherry tomatoes
- 1 tablespoon of tomato paste
- 3 garlic cloves, smashed and peeled
- ½-lb. of cremini mushroom, quartered
- 2 medium carrot, chopped coarsely
- 1 small onion, chopped coarsely
- 1 teaspoon of olive oil
- 6 boneless, skinless chicken thighs

DIRECTIONS

1. Place a heavy-bottomed pot on medium-high fire and heat the pot for 3 minutes.
2. Meanwhile, season chicken generously with pepper.
3. Once hot, add oil and stir around to coat the pot with oil.
4. Pan Fry chicken for 4 minutes per side and transfer to a plate.
5. Add the mushrooms, carrots, and onions to the pot. Season with pepper. Sauté for 5 minutes.
6. Add the tomato paste and garlic. Sauté for 2 minutes.
7. Add the olives, cherry tomatoes, and return the chicken. Mix well.
8. Cover, bring to a boil, lower the fire to a simmer, and simmer for 10 minutes.
9. Stir in the fresh herbs.
10. Serve and enjoy.

NUTRITION

- Calories: 241
- Carbs: 7.7 g
- Protein: 21.5 g
- Fat: 13.9 g
- Saturated Fat: 3.7 g
- Sodium: 403 mg

ITALIAN CHICKEN CACCIATORE

Preparation Time: 10 minutes
Cooking Time: 30-40minutes
Servings: 2

INGREDIENTS

- ¼ cup of balsamic vinegar
- 1 teaspoon of fresh thyme
- 2 tablespoon of parsley
- 1 14.5-oz. of can low sodium diced tomatoes, pulsed in a blender
- 1 14.5-oz. of can low sodium diced tomatoes in juice
- 1 cup of chicken broth
- 1 bay leaf
- 2 tablespoon of fresh basil, chopped
- ¼ teaspoon of red pepper flakes
- 1 teaspoon of dried oregano
- 2 large garlic cloves, minced
- ½-lb. of mushrooms, sliced
- 1 red bell pepper, diced
- 3 carrots, peeled and diced
- 1 medium onion, sliced thinly
- 1 tablespoon of extra virgin olive oil
- 2 teaspoon of ground pepper
- 6 chicken thighs, pat dry with paper towels

DIRECTIONS

1. Place a heavy-bottomed pot on medium-high fire and heat the pot for 3 minutes.
2. Meanwhile, season the chicken generously with pepper.
3. Once hot, add the oil and stir around to coat the pot with oil.
4. Brown the chicken for 5 minutes per side. If needed, cook in batches and place on a plate.
5. Add the mushroom and onion. Sauté for 5 minutes.
6. Stir in pepper flakes, oregano, and garlic. Cook for a minute.
7. Stir in thyme and bay leaf. Cook for another minute.
8. Pour in the tomatoes, chicken broth, bell pepper, carrots, and the chicken. Mix well.
9. Cover, bring to a boil, lower the fire to a simmer, and simmer for 10 minutes.
10. Serve and enjoy with a sprinkle of parsley.

NUTRITION

- Calories: 412
- Carbs: 43 g
- Protein: 37 g
- Fat: 13 g
- Saturated Fat: 3.6 g
- Sodium: 364 mg

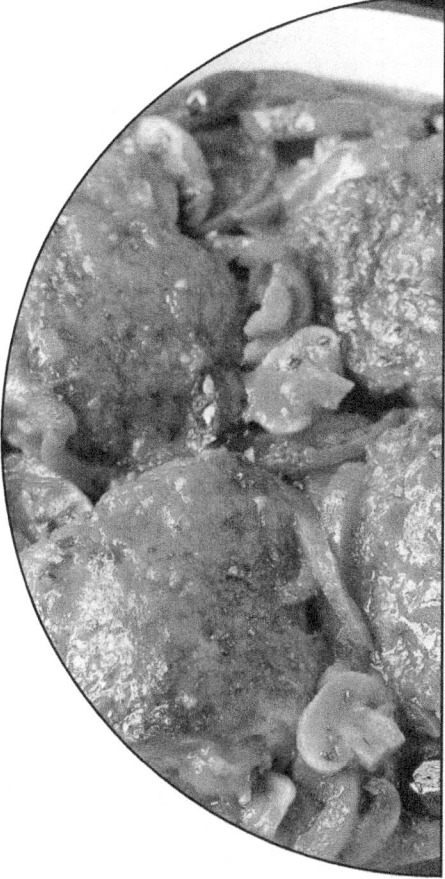

OREGANO-BASIL CHICKEN BREAST

Preparation Time: 10 minutes
Cooking Time: 25 minutes
Servings: 2

INGREDIENTS

- 1/2 cup of water
- 1/8 teaspoon of dried basil
- 1/8 teaspoon of dried oregano
- 2 tablespoon of balsamic vinegar
- Black pepper to taste
- 2 boneless, skinless chicken breasts
- 1 tablespoon of oil

DIRECTIONS

1. Place a heavy-bottomed pot on medium-high fire and heat the pot for 3 minutes.
2. Meanwhile, season chicken generously with pepper.
3. Once hot, add oil and stir around to coat the pot with oil.
4. Add the chicken breasts to hot pot and cook for 5 minutes per side.
5. Add the remaining ingredients to the pot.
6. Cover, bring to a boil, lower the fire to a simmer, and simmer for 10 minutes.
7. Serve and enjoy.

NUTRITION

- Calories: 142
- Carbs: 2.5 g
- Protein: 19.1 g
- Fat: 5.8 g
- Saturated Fat: 1.0 g
- Sodium: 305 mg

FILIPINO STYLE CHICKEN ADOBO

Preparation Time: 10 minutes
Cooking Time: 35 minutes
Servings: 2

INGREDIENTS

- 4 dried bay leaves
- 1 teaspoon of ground black peppercorn
- 1 large sweet onion, chopped
- 10 cloves of garlic, smashed
- ¼ cup of vinegar
- 2 tablespoon of coconut aminos
- 1.5-lbs of chicken breast, boneless and skinless, cut into 2-inch cubes

DIRECTIONS

1. Place a heavy-bottomed pot on medium-high fire and heat the pot for 3 minutes.
2. Once hot, add oil and stir around to coat the pot with oil.
3. Add the garlic and sauté for 2 minutes or until lightly browned.
4. Add half of the onions and sauté until soft, around 4 minutes.
5. Stir in chicken and cook for 10 minutes.
6. Add the remaining ingredients, except for onions.
7. Cover, bring to a boil, lower the fire to a simmer, and simmer for 15 minutes.
8. Stir in the remaining onions.
9. Serve and enjoy.

NUTRITION

- Calories: 169
- Carbs: 3.1 g
- Protein: 23.5 g
- Fat: 6.3 g
- Saturated Fat: 1.8 g
- Sodium: 328 mg

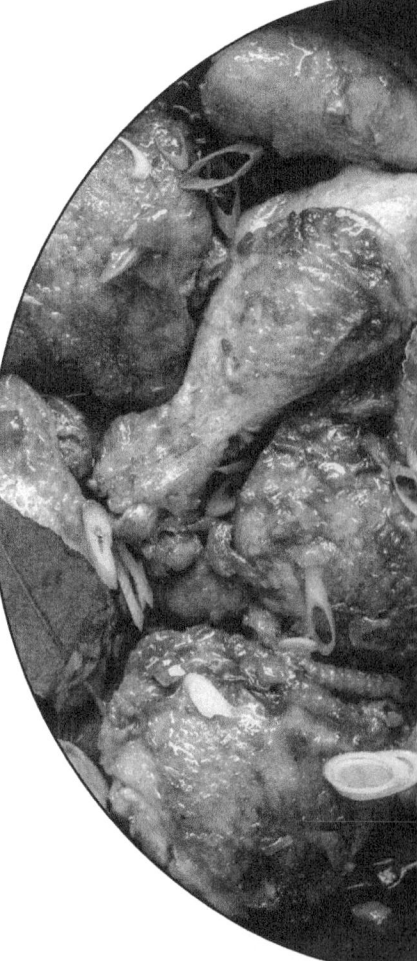

STEWED CHICKEN & DRIED CHERRIES

Preparation Time: 10 minutes
Cooking Time: 25 minutes
Servings: 2

INGREDIENTS

- 1 tablespoon of olive oil
- 1 cup of shredded chicken meat
- 1 onion, chopped
- 2 teaspoons of chili powder
- 1 teaspoon of sambal oelek
- 1 tablespoon of coconut aminos
- 2 cans of cannellini beans, drained and rinsed
- ½ cup of dried cherries
- 2 cups of chicken broth, low sodium
- Pepper to taste
- 2 tablespoons of chopped parsley

DIRECTIONS

1. Place a heavy-bottomed pot on medium-high fire and heat the pot for 3 minutes.
2. Once hot, add oil and stir around to coat the pot with oil. Sauté the chicken meat, onions, chili powder, and sambal oelek for 5 minutes. Season with coconut aminos.
3. Stir in the cannellini beans and cherries.
4. Add the broth and season with pepper.
5. Cover, bring to a boil, lower the fire to a simmer, and simmer for 15 minutes.
6. Serve and enjoy with a sprinkle of parsley.

NUTRITION

- Calories: 278
- Carbs: 33.1 g
- Protein: 16.8 g
- Fat: 9.0 g
- Saturated Fat: 1.6 g
- Sodium: 264 mg

CHICKEN 'N GINGER CONGEE

Preparation Time: 10 minutes
Cooking Time: 45 minutes
Servings: 2

INGREDIENTS

- 8 cups of water
- 3 boneless chicken thighs, sliced thinly
- 1 cup of rice, uncooked
- 4 thick slices of ginger, smashed
- ½ teaspoon of salt
- 4 cloves garlic, peeled and minced
- ½ cup of scallions, chopped
- 3 tablespoons of ginger, minced
- ½ cup of cilantro leaves
- 1 teaspoon of olive oil
- Pepper to taste

DIRECTIONS

1. Place a heavy-bottomed pot on medium-high fire and heat pot for 3 minutes.
2. Meanwhile, season the chicken generously with pepper.
3. Once hot, add oil and stir around to coat the pot with oil.
4. Sauté garlic and ginger for 3 minutes. Add the chicken and sauté for 3 minutes.
5. Add 4 cups of water and the remaining ingredients except for cilantro and scallions. Mix well.
6. Cover, bring to a boil and boil for 5 minutes.
7. Stir in the remaining water; bring to a simmer for 25 minutes. Continue cooking until rice is soft and tender.
8. Stir in the cilantro.
9. Serve and enjoy with a sprinkle of pepper and scallions.

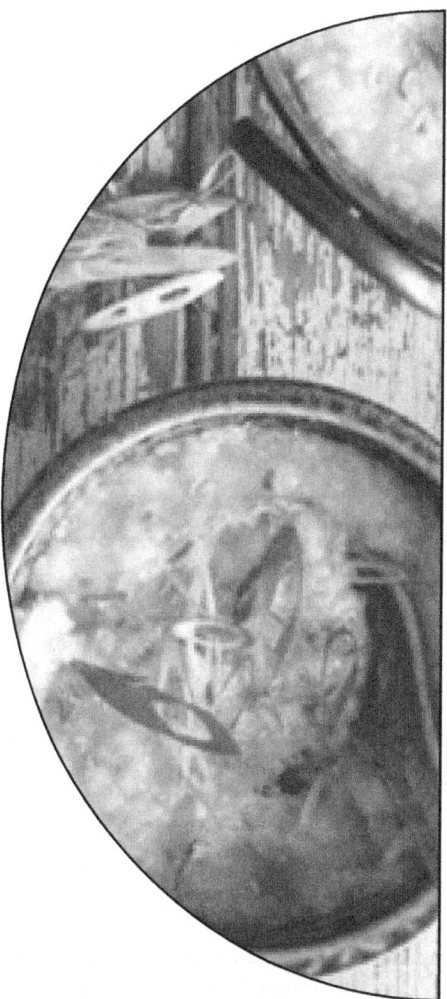

BROCCOLI-CHICKEN RICE

Preparation Time: 10 minutes
Cooking Time: 35 minutes
Servings: 2

INGREDIENTS

- 1 teaspoon of olive oil
- 1-pound of boneless chicken breasts, sliced thinly
- 2 cloves of garlic, minced
- 1 onion, chopped
- Pepper to taste
- 1 1/3 cups of long-grain rice
- 1 1/3 cups of chicken broth, low sodium
- ½ cup of skim milk
- 1 cup of broccoli florets
- ½ cup of low-fat cheddar cheese, grated

DIRECTIONS

1. Place a heavy-bottomed pot on medium-high fire and heat the pot for 3 minutes.
2. Meanwhile, season the chicken generously with pepper.
3. Once hot, add oil and stir around to coat the pot with oil.
4. Sauté the garlic and onion for 3 minutes. Add the chicken and cook for another 3 minutes.
5. Add the rice and stir-fry for 3 minutes.
6. Stir in the chicken broth and season with pepper. Cover and simmer for 10 minutes or until water is fully absorbed.
7. Add the broccoli florets and skim milk. Cover and simmer for another 5 minutes.
8. Sprinkle cheese on top, cover and let it sit for 5 minutes.
9. Serve and enjoy.

RANCH RISOTTO

Preparation Time: 40 minutes
Cooking Time: 30 minutes
Servings: 2

INGREDIENTS

- 1 onion, diced
- 2 cups of chicken stock, boiling
- ½ cup of parmesan OR cheddar cheese, grated
- 1 clove garlic, minced
- ¾ cup of Arborio rice
- 1 tablespoon of olive oil
- 1 tablespoon of unsalted butter

DIRECTIONS

1. Set the Air Fryer at 390 °F for 5 minutes to heat up.
2. With oil, grease a round baking tin, small enough to fit inside the fryer, and stir in the garlic, butter, and onion.
3. Transfer the tin to the Air Fryer and allow cooking for 4 minutes. Add in the rice and cook for a further 4 minutes, stirring it three times throughout the cooking time.
4. Turn the fryer down to 320 °F and add in the chicken stock before gently mixing it. Leave to cook for 22 minutes with the fryer uncovered. Before serving, throw in the cheese and give it one more stir. Enjoy!

NUTRITION
- Calories: 239
- Fat: 11.5 g
- Fiber: 3.4 g
- Carbs: 11.5 g
- Protein: 5.6 g

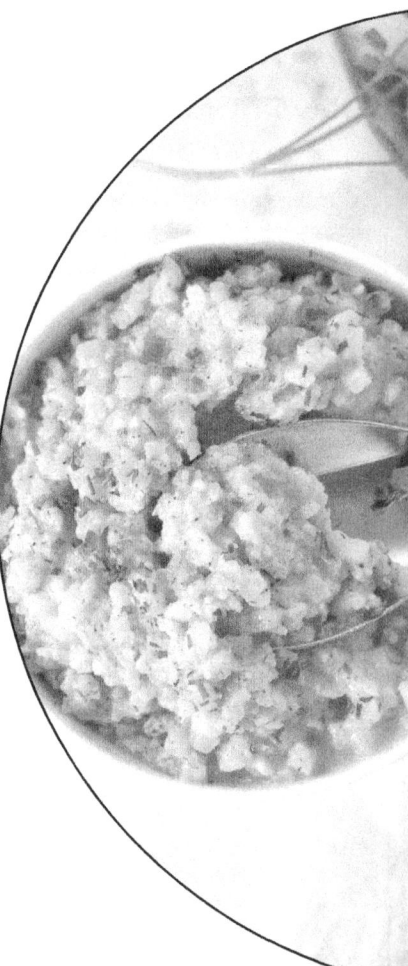

STEWED CHICKEN & DRIED CHERRIES

Preparation Time: 10 minutes
Cooking Time: 25 minutes
Servings: 2

INGREDIENTS

- 1 tablespoon of olive oil
- 1 cup of shredded chicken meat
- 1 onion, chopped
- 2 teaspoons of chili powder
- 1 teaspoon of sambal oelek
- 1 tablespoon of coconut aminos
- 2 cans of cannellini beans, drained and rinsed
- ½ cup of dried cherries
- 2 cups of chicken broth, low sodium
- Pepper to taste
- 2 tablespoons of chopped parsley

DIRECTIONS

1. Place a heavy-bottomed pot on medium-high fire and heat the pot for 3 minutes.
2. Once hot, add oil and stir around to coat the pot with oil. Sauté the chicken meat, onions, chili powder, and sambal oelek for 5 minutes. Season with coconut aminos.
3. Stir in the cannellini beans and cherries.
4. Add the broth and season with pepper.
5. Cover, bring to a boil, lower the fire to a simmer, and simmer for 15 minutes.
6. Serve and enjoy with a sprinkle of parsley.

NUTRITION
- Calories: 278
- Carbs: 33.1 g
- Protein: 16.8 g
- Fat: 9.0 g
- Saturated Fat: 1.6 g
- Sodium: 264 mg

CHAPTER 5.
MEAT

SPICY BEEF CURRY

Preparation Time: 15 minutes
Cooking Time: 40 minutes
Servings: 2

INGREDIENTS

- ½ pound of lean ground beef
- ¾ cup of chopped onion
- ½ cup of bell pepper, any color, seeded and chopped
- ½ tablespoon of chili powder
- 1 tablespoon of oregano
- 1 cup of tomatoes, chopped
- 1 cup of frozen vegetable mix, chopped
- 2 cups of water
- 1/2 cup of shredded Mexican cheese blend

DIRECTIONS

1. Place the beef in a large skillet and add onions. Sauté for 3 minutes or until the beef has slightly rendered its fat.
2. Stir in the bell pepper, chili powder, and oregano and cook for another minute.
3. Add in the tomatoes, vegetable mix and water.
4. Close the lid and bring it to a simmer for 10 minutes.
5. Before serving, stir in cheese.

NUTRITION

- Calories: 222
- Protein: 20 g
- Carbs: 11 g
- Fat: 10 g
- Saturated Fat: 5 g
- Sodium: 132 mg

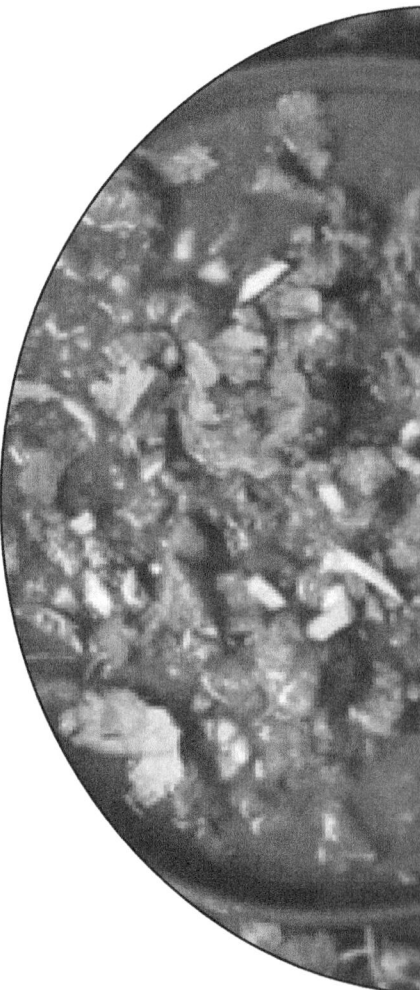

PORK TENDERLOIN WITH APPLES AND SWEET POTATOES

Preparation Time: 15 minutes
Cooking Time: 30 minutes
Servings: 2

INGREDIENTS

- ¾ cup of apple cider
- ¼ cup of apple cider vinegar
- 2 tablespoons of maple syrup
- ¼ teaspoon of smoked paprika powder
- 1 teaspoon of grated ginger
- ¼ teaspoon of ground black pepper
- 2 teaspoons of olive oil
- 1 12-ounces of pork tenderloin
- 1 large sweet potato, cut into cubes
- 1 large apple, cored and into cubes

DIRECTIONS

1. Preheat the oven to 375 ºF.
2. In a bowl, combine the apple cider, apple cider vinegar, maple syrup, smoked paprika, ginger, and black pepper. Set aside.
3. Heat the oil in a large skillet and sear the meat for 3 minutes on both sides.
4. Transfer the pork to a baking dish and place the sweet potatoes and apples around the pork. Pour in the apple cider sauce.
5. Place inside the oven and cook for 20 minutes.

NUTRITION

- Calories: 267
- Protein: 23.5 g
- Carbs: 31 g
- Fat: 5 g
- Saturated Fat: 0.5 g
- Sodium: 69 mg

MEXICAN BEEF AND VEGGIE SKILLET

Preparation Time: 15 minutes
Cooking Time: 15 minutes
Servings: 2

INGREDIENTS

- 2 lbs. beef
- 1 medium Serrano pepper, cut into thirds
- 4 cloves of garlic, minced
- 1 2-inch of piece ginger, peeled and chopped
- 1 yellow onion, chopped
- 2 tablespoon of ground coriander
- 2 teaspoons of ground cumin
- ½ teaspoon of ground turmeric
- 2 teaspoons of garam masala
- 1 tablespoon of olive oil
- pounds of beef, cut into chunks
- 1 cup of ripe tomatoes, diced
- 2 cups of water
- 1 cup of fresh cilantro for garnish

DIRECTIONS

1. In a food processor, pulse the Serrano peppers, garlic, ginger, onion, coriander, cumin, turmeric, and garam masala until well combined.
2. Heat oil over medium heat in a skillet and sauté the spice mixture for 2 minutes or until fragrant.
3. Stir in the beef and cook constantly stirring for 3 minutes or until the meat turns brown.
4. Stir in the tomatoes and sauté for another 3 minutes.
5. Add in the water and bring to a boil.
6. Once boiling, turn the heat to low and simmer for thirty minutes or until the meat is tender.
7. Add the cilantro last before serving.

NUTRITION

- Calories: 181
- Protein: 16 g
- Carbs: 5 g
- Fat: 8 g
- Saturated Fat: 2 g
- Sodium: 74 mg

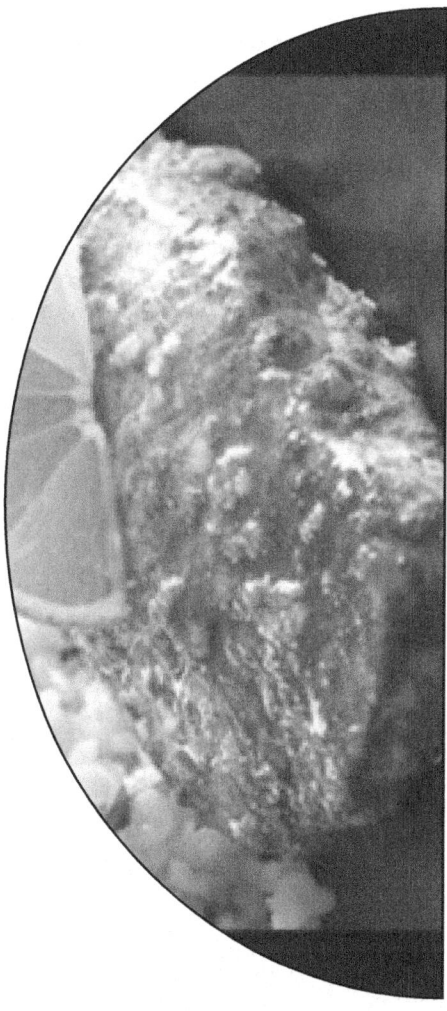

GARLIC LIME MARINATED PORK CHOPS

Preparation Time: 15 minutes
Cooking Time: 10 minutes
Servings: 2

INGREDIENTS

- 4 6-ounces of lean boneless pork chops, trimmed from fat
- 4 cloves of garlic, crushed
- 1 teaspoon of cumin
- 1 teaspoon of chili powder
- 1 teaspoon of paprika
- A dash of black pepper to taste
- Juice from ½ lime
- Zest from ½ lime

DIRECTIONS

1. In a bowl, season the pork with the rest of the ingredients.
2. Allow marinating inside the fridge for at least 2 hours.
3. Place the pork chops in a baking dish or broiler pan and grill for 5 minutes on each side until golden brown.
4. Serve with salad if desired.

NUTRITION

- Calories: 233
- Protein: 38.5 g
- Carbs: 4 g
- Fat: 6 g
- Saturated Fat: 1 g
- Sodium: 105 mg

ORIENTAL STIR FRY

Preparation Time: 15 minutes
Cooking Time: 20 minutes
Servings: 2

INGREDIENTS

- 4 ounces of pork loin, cut into thin strips
- 1 tablespoon of ginger, minced
- 1 clove of garlic, chopped
- 1 ½ cups of sliced onions
- 1 medium carrot, sliced thinly
- 2 medium green bell peppers, seeded and cut into thick strips
- 1 cup of sliced celery
- 1 cup of dried plums, pitted and halved
- 2 tablespoons of low sodium soy sauce
- ¼ cup of cold water + 2 tablespoons of cornstarch

DIRECTIONS

1. In a skillet, sauté the pork on medium heat until it has slightly rendered fat.
2. Stir in the ginger, garlic, and onions until fragrant.
3. Stir in the carrots, green bell peppers, celery, and plums.
4. Season with soy sauce.
5. Close the lid and adjust the flame to low. Cook for 10 minutes while stirring every 3 minutes.
6. Open the lid and adjust the flame to medium. Stir in the cornstarch slurry and cook for another 5 minutes until the sauce thickens.

NUTRITION

- Calories: 145
- Protein: 9 g
- Carbs: 21 g
- Fat: 3 g
- Saturated Fat: 0.4 g
- Sodium: 106 mg

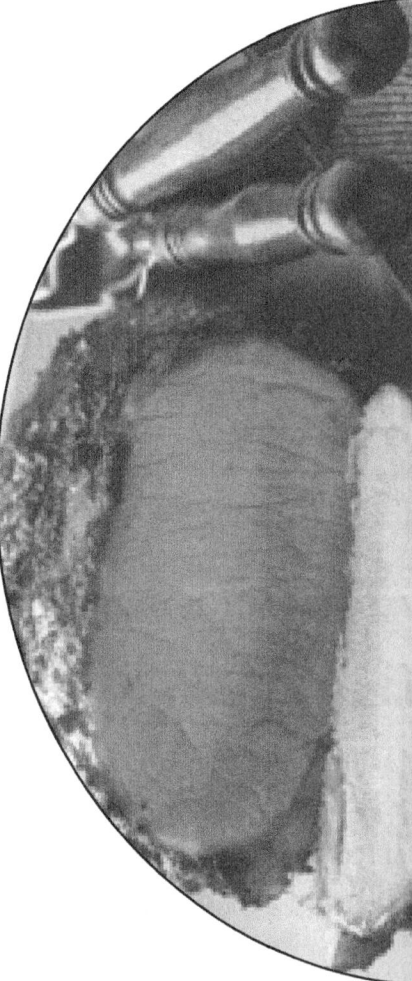

COCOA-CRUSTED PORK TENDERLOIN

Preparation Time: 15 minutes
Cooking Time: 25 minutes
Servings: 2

INGREDIENTS

- 1-pound of pork tenderloin, trimmed from fat
- 1 tablespoon of cocoa powder
- 1 teaspoon of instant coffee powder
- ½ teaspoon of ground cinnamon
- ½ teaspoon of chili powder
- 1 tablespoon of olive oil

DIRECTIONS

1. In a bowl, dust the pork tenderloin with cocoa powder, coffee, cinnamon, and chili powder.
2. In a skillet, heat the oil and sear the meat for 5 minutes on both sides over low to medium flame.
3. Transfer the pork to a baking dish and cook in the oven for 15 minutes in a 350 °F preheated oven.

NUTRITION

- Calories: 395
- Protein: 60 g
- Carbs: 2 g
- Fat: 15 g
- Saturated Fat: 4 g
- Sodium: 150 mg

BEEF KABOBS WITH PINEAPPLES

Preparation Time: 15 minutes
Cooking Time: 10 minutes
Servings: 2

INGREDIENTS

- 1 ½ pound of beef shoulder steaks, cut into thick chunks
- A dash of ground black pepper
- 2 tablespoons of olive oil
- 2 tablespoons of lime juice
- 2 cloves of garlic, minced
- ½ teaspoon of ground cumin
- 1 cup of pineapple chunks
- 12 wooden skewers, soaked in water for 30 minutes

DIRECTIONS

1. In a bowl, combine the beef, black pepper, olive oil, lime juice, garlic, and cumin until well incorporated.
2. Place inside the fridge and allow marinating for at least 3 hours.
3. Thread one chunk of beef and a chunk of pineapple alternately through the wooden skewer. Do two or three alternating layers.
4. Heat the grill to 350 ºF and place the grill rack 6 inches away from the charcoal.
5. Grill the kabobs for 5 minutes on each side.

NUTRITION
- Calories: 243
- Protein: 24 g
- Carbs: 11 g
- Fat: 11 g
- Saturated Fat: 1 g
- Sodium: 71 mg

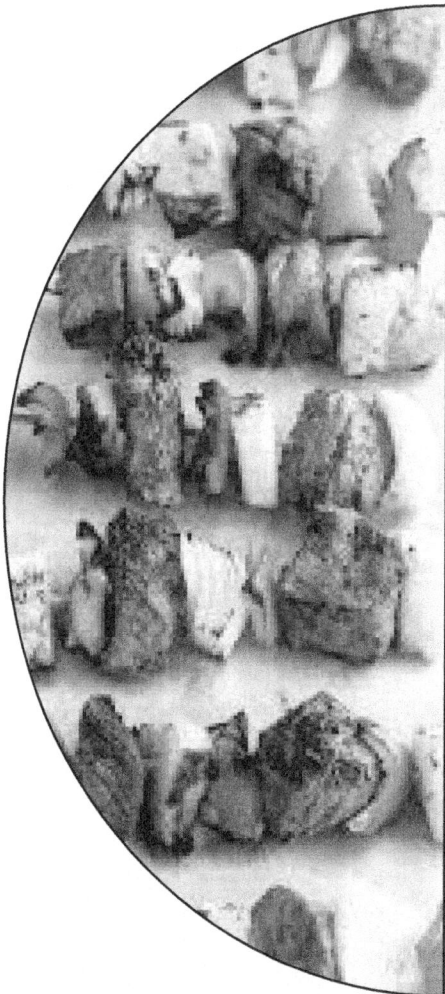

ASIAN BEEF AND ZUCCHINI NOODLES

Preparation Time: 15 minutes
Cooking Time: 15 minutes
Servings: 2

INGREDIENTS

- ½ pound of lean ground beef
- 1 tablespoon of minced ginger
- 2 cloves of garlic, minced
- 16 ounces Asian-style vegetable package, frozen
- 2 cups of low sodium beef broth
- 1 large zucchini, spiralized or thinly sliced
- 2 green onions, sliced thinly

DIRECTIONS

1. In a large skillet, sauté the beef with minced ginger and garlic for 3 minutes while constantly stirring.
2. Stir in the vegetable package and the beef broth.
3. Bring to a boil for 10 minutes.
4. Assemble the dish by putting the zucchini in a bowl.
5. Pour in the soup and garnish with green onions.

NUTRITION
- Calories: 271
- Protein: 23 g
- Carbs: 21 g
- Fat: 5 g
- Saturated Fat: 3 g
- Sodium: 138 mg

EXOTIC THAI STEAK

Preparation Time: 15 minutes
Cooking Time: 20 minutes
Servings: 2

INGREDIENTS

- 1-pound of London broil, trimmed from fat
- 2 tablespoons of light fish sauce
- 1 tablespoon of olive oil
- 2 cloves of garlic, minced
- ½ teaspoon of grated ginger
- ½ cup of chopped coriander
- ¼ cup of white vinegar
- 2 tablespoons of honey

DIRECTIONS

1. Place in a Ziploc bag all the ingredients and marinate in the fridge for at least 3 hours.
2. Heat the grill to low heat.
3. Place the meat on the grill rack and cook for 10 minutes on each side or until the internal temperature reaches 175 °F.
4. Slice the London broil and serve with vegetables.

NUTRITION

- Calories: 219
- Protein: 23 g
- Carbs: 9 g
- Fat: 5 g
- Saturated Fat: 1 g
- Sodium: 100 mg

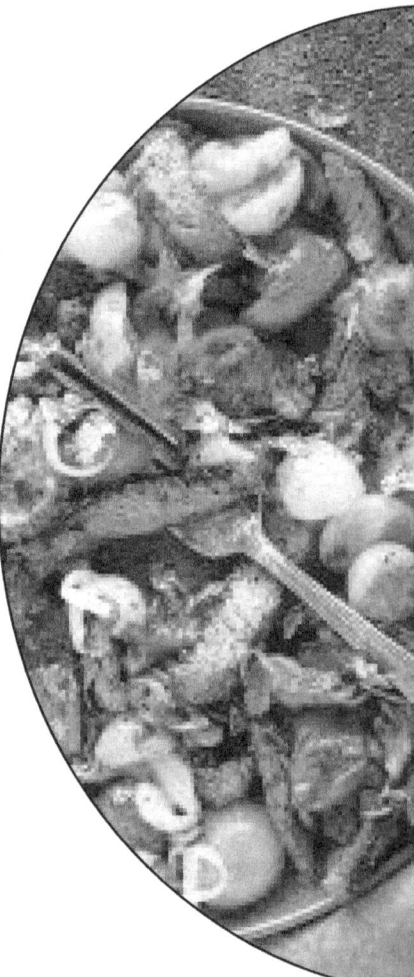

SWEET AND SPICY EDAMAME BEEF STEW

Preparation Time: 15 minutes
Cooking Time: 20 minutes
Servings: 2

INGREDIENTS

- 1 tablespoon of olive oil
- 8 ounces of sirloin steak, trimmed from fat
- 2 teaspoon of ginger, finely chopped
- 3 cloves of garlic, minced
- 3 cups of packaged vegetable of your choice
- 1 cup of shelled sweet soybeans or edamame
- 3 tablespoons of hoisin sauce
- 2 tablespoons of rice vinegar
- 1 teaspoon of red chili paste

DIRECTIONS

1. In a non-stick pan, heat the oil over medium flame.
2. Sauté the sirloin steak for 3 minutes while constantly stirring.
3. Stir in the ginger and garlic and sauté for 1 minute.
4. Add in the rest of the ingredients.
5. Close the lid and allow simmering for 10 minutes until the vegetables are cooked.

NUTRITION

- Calories: 205
- Protein: 14 g
- Carbs: 17 g
- Fat: 4 g
- Saturated Fat: 1 g
- Sodium: 146 mg

FILLING SIRLOIN SOUP

Preparation Time: 15 minutes
Cooking Time: 15 minutes
Servings: 2

INGREDIENTS

- 1 tablespoon of oil
- 1 small onion, diced
- 3 cloves of garlic, minced
- 1-pound of lean ground sirloin
- 3 cups of low sodium beef broth
- 1 bag of frozen vegetables of your choice
- Black pepper to taste

DIRECTIONS

1. In a large saucepan, heat the oil over medium heat and sauté the onion and garlic until fragrant.
2. Stir in the lean ground sirloin and cook for 3 minutes until lightly golden.
3. Add in the rest of the ingredients and bring the broth to a boil for 10 minutes.
4. Serve warm.

NUTRITION

- Calories: 245
- Protein: 29 g
- Carbs: 22 g
- Fat: 4 g
- Saturated Fat: 1 g
- Sodium: 152 mg

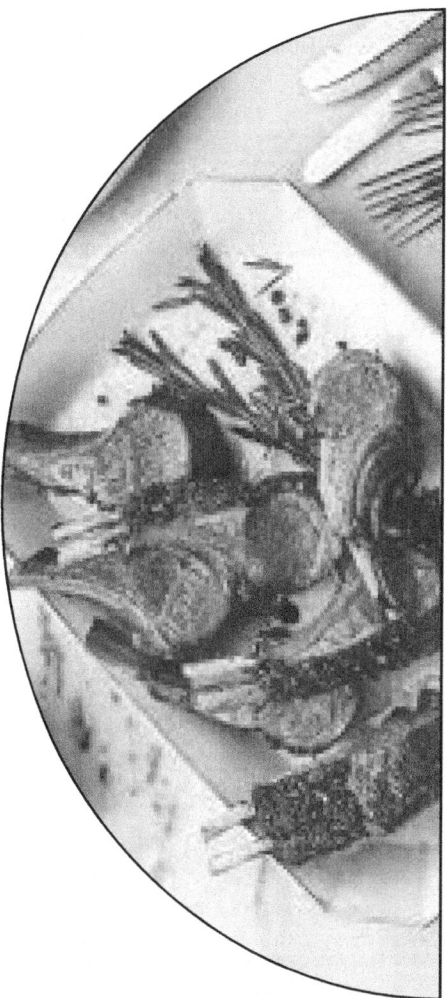

ROAST RACK OF LAMB

Preparation Time: 15 minutes
Cooking Time: 30 minutes
Servings: 2

INGREDIENTS

- 2 1-pound of French-style lamb rib roast, trimmed from fat
- 1 cup of dry red wine
- 2 cloves of garlic, minced
- 1 teaspoon of freshly grated nutmeg
- 1 tablespoon of olive oil
- 1 tablespoon of chopped rosemary
- 3 tablespoons of dried cranberries, chopped

DIRECTIONS

1. In a resealable plastic, place the lamb and add red wine, garlic, nutmeg, olive oil, and rosemary. Seal the bag and turn it to coat the lamb with the spices. Marinate inside the fridge for at least 4 hours while turning the bag occasionally.
2. Preheat the oven to 450 °F and remove the lamb from the marinade. Reserve the juices.
3. Place the lamb bone side down on a roasting pan lined with foil.
4. Pour the reserved marinade over the roasting pan.
5. Roast for 30 minutes until the lamb turns slightly golden. Turn the lamb every 10 minutes and baste it with the sauce.
6. Once cooked, take out the lamb from the oven and slice.
7. Serve with chopped cranberries on top.

NUTRITION

- Calories: 241
- Protein: 25 g
- Carbs: 1 g
- Fat: 12 g
- Saturated Fat: 3 g
- Sodium: 46 mg

GARLIC PORK MIX

Preparation Time: 10 minutes
Cooking Time: 45 minutes
Servings: 2

INGREDIENTS

- 2 pounds of pork meat, boneless and cubed
- 1 red onion, chopped
- 1 tablespoon of olive oil
- 3 garlic of cloves, minced
- 1 cup of low-sodium beef stock
- 2 tablespoons of sweet paprika
- Black pepper to the taste
- 1 tablespoon of chives, chopped

DIRECTIONS

1. Heat a pan with the oil over medium heat, add the onion and the meat, toss and brown for 5 minutes.
2. Add the rest of the ingredients, toss, reduce heat to medium, cover and cook for 40 minutes.
3. Divide the mix between plates and serve.

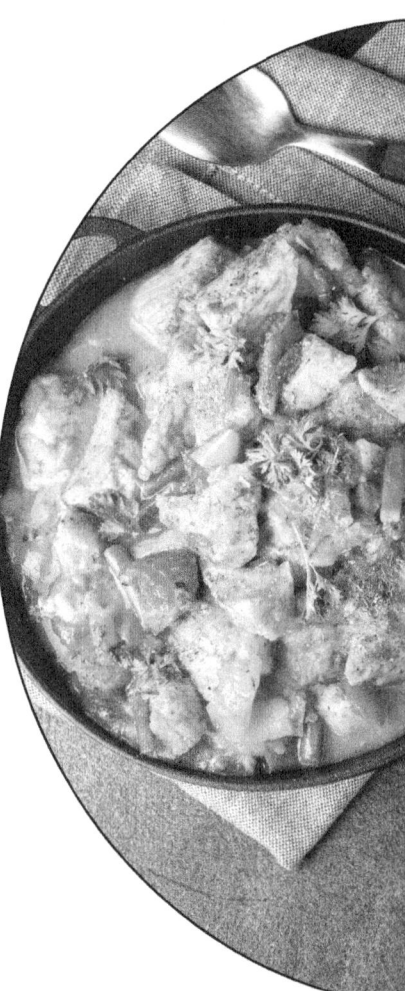

PAPRIKA PORK WITH CARROTS

Preparation Time: 10 minutes
Cooking Time: 30 minutes
Servings: 2

INGREDIENTS

- 1 pound of pork stew meat, cubed
- ¼ cup of low-sodium veggie stock
- 2 carrots, peeled and sliced
- 2 tablespoons of olive oil
- 1 red onion, sliced
- 2 teaspoons of sweet paprika
- Black pepper to the taste

DIRECTIONS

1. Heat a pan with the oil over medium heat; add the onion, stir and sauté for 5 minutes.
2. Add the meat, toss and brown for 5 minutes more.
3. Add the rest of the ingredients, bring to a simmer and cook over medium heat for 20 minutes.
4. Divide the mix between plates and serve.

GINGER PORK AND ONIONS

Preparation Time: 10 minutes
Cooking Time: 35 minutes
Servings: 2

INGREDIENTS

- 2 red onions, sliced
- 2 green onions, chopped
- 1 tablespoon of olive oil
- 2 teaspoons of ginger, grated
- 4 pork of chops
- 3 garlic cloves, chopped
- Black pepper to the taste
- 1 carrot, chopped
- 1 cup of low sodium beef stock
- 2 tablespoons of tomato paste
- 1 tablespoon of cilantro, chopped

DIRECTIONS

1. Heat a pan with the oil over medium heat, add the green and red onions, toss and sauté them for 3 minutes.
2. Add the garlic and the ginger, toss and cook for 2 minutes more.
3. Add the pork chops and cook them for 2 minutes on each side.
4. Add the rest of the ingredients, bring to a simmer and cook over medium heat for 25 minutes more.
5. Divide the mix between plates and serve.

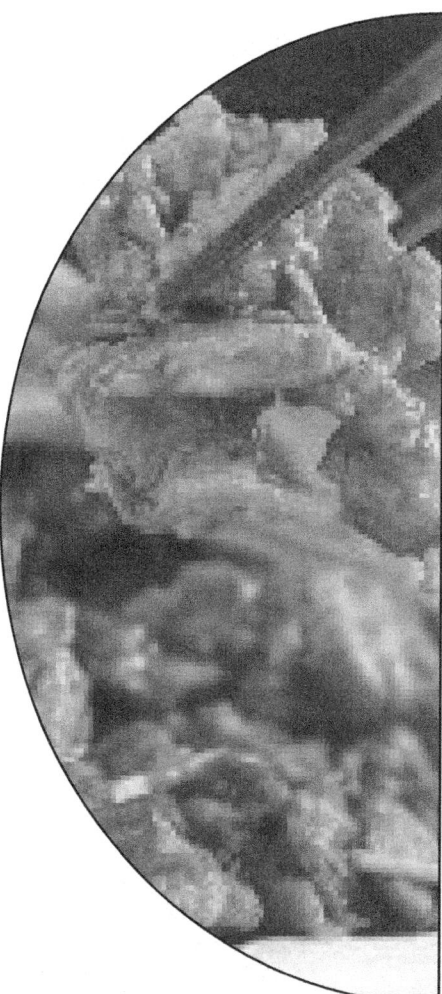

CUMIN PORK

Preparation Time: 10 minutes
Cooking Time: 45 minutes
Servings: 2

INGREDIENTS

- ½ cup of low-sodium beef stock
- 2 tablespoons of olive oil
- 2 pounds of pork stew meat, cubed
- 1 teaspoon of coriander, ground
- 2 teaspoons of cumin, ground
- Black pepper to the taste
- 1 cup of cherry tomatoes, halved
- 4 garlic cloves, minced
- 1 tablespoon of cilantro, chopped

DIRECTIONS

1. Heat a pan with the oil over medium heat, add the garlic and the meat, toss and brown for 5 minutes.
2. Add the stock and the other ingredients bring to a simmer and cook over medium heat for 40 minutes.
3. Divide everything between plates and serve.

PORK AND GREENS MIX

Preparation Time: 10 minutes
Cooking Time: 20 minutes
Servings: 2

INGREDIENTS

- 2 tablespoons of balsamic vinegar
- 1/3 cup of coconut aminos
- 1 tablespoon of olive oil
- 4 ounces of mixed salad greens
- 1 cup of cherry tomatoes, halved
- 4 ounces of pork stew meat, cut into strips
- 1 tablespoon of chives, chopped

DIRECTIONS

1. Heat a pan with the oil over medium heat, add the pork, aminos, vinegar, toss and cook for 15 minutes.
2. Add the salad greens and the other ingredients, toss, cook for 5 minutes more, divide between plates and serve.

NUTRITION

- Calories: 125
- Fat: 6.4 g
- Fiber: 0.6 g
- Carbs: 6.8 g
- Protein: 9.1 g

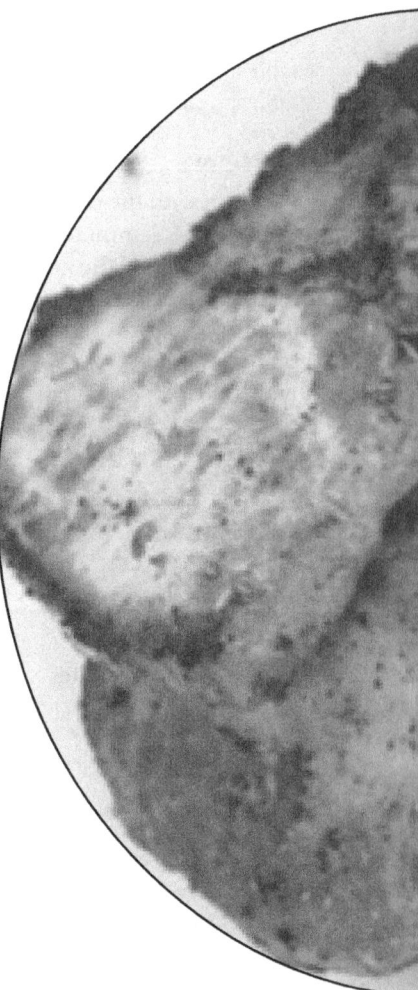

THYME PORK PAN

Preparation Time: 10 minutes
Cooking Time: 25 minutes
Servings: 2

INGREDIENTS

- 1 pound of pork butt, trimmed and cubed
- 1 tablespoon of olive oil
- 1 yellow onion, chopped
- 3 garlic cloves, minced
- 1 tablespoon of thyme, dried
- 1 cup of low-sodium chicken stock
- 2 tablespoons of low-sodium tomato paste
- 1 tablespoon of cilantro, chopped

DIRECTIONS

1. Heat a pan with the oil over medium-high heat, add the onion and the garlic, toss and cook for 5 minutes.
2. Add the meat, toss and cook for 5 more minutes.
3. Add the rest of the ingredients, toss, bring to a simmer, reduce heat to medium and cook the mix for 15 minutes more.
4. Divide the mix between plates and serve right away.

NUTRITION

- Calories: 281
- Fat: 11.2 g
- Fiber: 1.4 g
- Carbs: 6.8 g
- Protein: 37.1 g

MARJORAM PORK AND ZUCCHINIS

Preparation Time: 10 minutes
Cooking Time: 30 minutes
Servings: 2

INGREDIENTS

- 2 pounds of pork loin boneless, trimmed and cubed
- 2 tablespoons of avocado oil
- ¾ cup of low-sodium veggie stock
- ½ tablespoon of garlic powder
- 1 tablespoon of marjoram, chopped
- 2 zucchinis, roughly cubed
- 1 teaspoon of sweet paprika
- Black pepper to the taste

DIRECTIONS

1. Heat a pan with the oil over medium-high heat, add the meat, garlic powder and marjoram, toss and cook for 10 minutes.
2. Add the zucchinis and the other ingredients toss, bring to a simmer, reduce heat to medium and cook the mix for 20 minutes more.
3. Divide everything between plates and serve.

NUTRITION

- Calories: 359
- Fat: 9.1 g
- Fiber: 2.1 g
- Carbs: 5.7 g
- Protein: 61.4 g

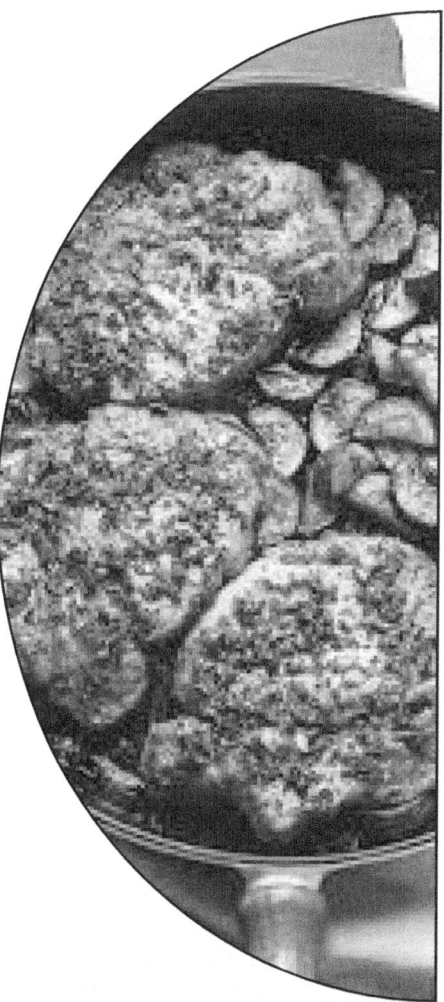

SPICED PORK

Preparation Time: 10 minutes
Cooking Time: 8 hours
Servings: 2

INGREDIENTS

- 3 tablespoons of olive oil
- 2 pounds of pork shoulder roast
- 2 teaspoons of sweet paprika
- 1 teaspoon of garlic powder
- 1 teaspoon of onion powder
- 1 teaspoon of nutmeg, ground
- 1 teaspoon of allspice, ground
- Black pepper to the taste
- 1 cup of low-sodium veggie stock

DIRECTIONS

1. In your slow cooker, combine the roast with the oil and the other ingredients, toss, put the lid on and cook on Low for 8 hours.
2. Slice the roast, divide it between plates and serve with the cooking juices drizzled on top.

NUTRITION

- Calories: 689
- Fat: 57.1 g
- Fiber: 1 g
- Carbs: 3.2 g
- Protein: 38.8 g

COCONUT PORK AND CELERY

Preparation Time: 10 minutes
Cooking Time: 35 minutes
Servings: 2

INGREDIENTS

- 2 pounds of pork stew meat, cubed
- 2 tablespoons of olive oil
- 1 cup of low-sodium veggie stock
- 1 celery stalk, chopped
- 1 teaspoon of black peppercorns
- 2 shallots, chopped
- 1 tablespoon of chives, chopped
- 1 cup of coconut cream
- Black pepper to the taste

DIRECTIONS

1. Heat a pan with the oil over medium heat, add the shallots and the meat, toss and brown for 5 minutes.
2. Add the celery and the other ingredients. Toss. Bring to a simmer and cook over medium heat for 30 minutes more.
3. Divide everything between plates and serve right away.

NUTRITION

- Calories: 690
- Fat: 43.3 g
- Fiber: 1.8 g
- Carbs: 5.7 g
- Protein: 6.2 g

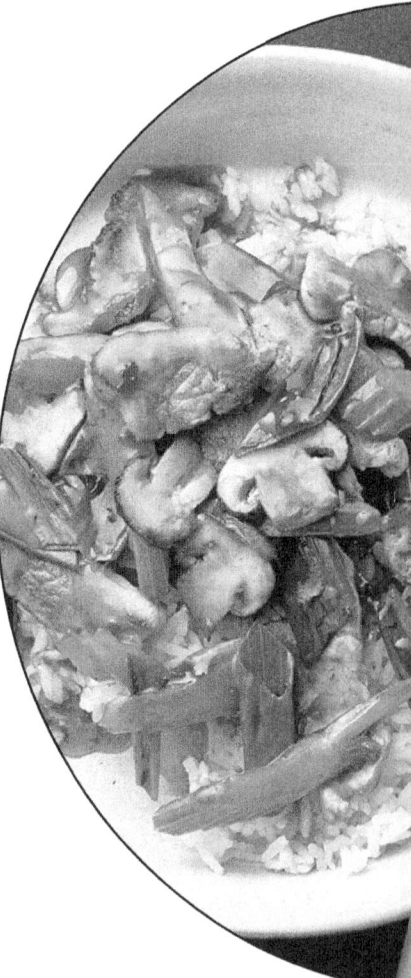

PORK AND TOMATOES MIX

Preparation Time: 10 minutes
Cooking Time: 30 minutes
Servings: 2

INGREDIENTS

- 2 garlic cloves, minced
- 2 pounds of pork stew meat, ground
- 2 cups of cherry tomatoes, halved
- 1 tablespoon of olive oil
- Black pepper to the taste
- 1 red onion, chopped
- ½ cup of low-sodium veggie stock
- 2 tablespoons of low-sodium tomato paste
- 1 tablespoon of parsley, chopped

DIRECTIONS

1. Heat a pan with the oil over medium heat; add the onion and the garlic, toss and sauté for 5 minutes.
2. Add the meat and brown it for 5 minutes more.
3. Add the rest of the ingredients, toss, bring to a simmer, cook over medium heat for 20 minutes more, divide into bowls and serve.

NUTRITION

- Calories: 558
- Fat: 25.6 g
- Fiber: 2.4 g
- Carbs: 10.1 g
- Protein: 68.7 g

SAGE PORK CHOPS

Preparation Time: 10 minutes
Cooking Time: 35 minutes
Servings: 2

INGREDIENTS

- 4 pork chops
- 2 tablespoons of olive oil
- 1 teaspoon of smoked paprika
- 1 tablespoon of sage, chopped
- 2 garlic cloves, minced
- 1 tablespoon of lemon juice
- Black pepper to the taste

DIRECTIONS

1. In a baking dish, combine the pork chops with the oil and the other ingredients, toss, introduce in the oven and bake at 400 °F for 35 minutes.
2. Divide the pork chops between plates and serve with a side salad.

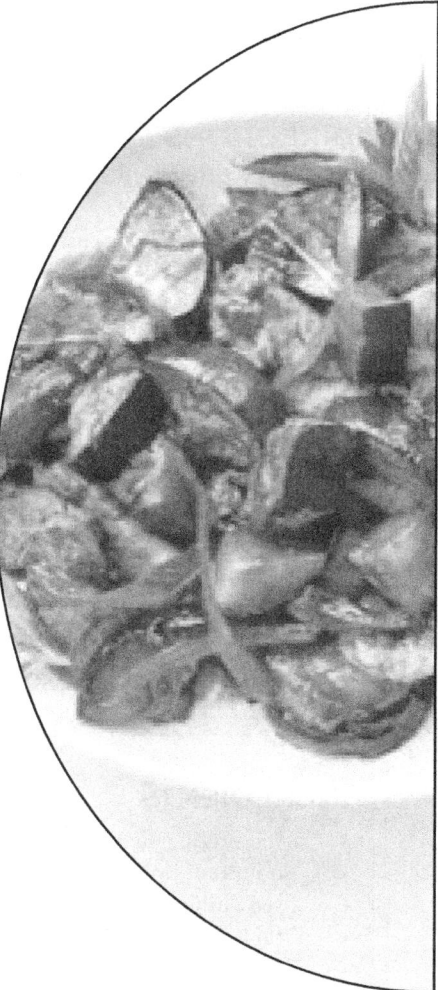

THAI PORK AND EGGPLANT

Preparation Time: 10 minutes
Cooking Time: 30 minutes
Servings: 2

INGREDIENTS

- 1 pound of pork stew meat, cubed
- 1 eggplant, cubed
- 1 tablespoon of coconut aminos
- 1 teaspoon of five-spice
- 2 garlic cloves, minced
- 2 Thai chilies, chopped
- 2 tablespoons of olive oil
- 2 tablespoons of low-sodium tomato paste
- 1 tablespoon of cilantro, chopped
- ½ cup of low-sodium veggie stock

DIRECTIONS

1. Heat a pan with the oil over medium-high heat and add the garlic, chilies, meat, and brown for 6 minutes.
2. Add the eggplant and the other ingredients bring to a simmer and cook over medium heat for 24 minutes.
3. Divide the mix between plates and serve.

PORK AND LIME SCALLIONS

Preparation Time: 10 minutes
Cooking Time: 30 minutes
Servings: 2

INGREDIENTS

- 2 tablespoons of lime juice
- 4 scallions, chopped
- 1 pound of pork stew meat, cubed
- 2 garlic cloves, minced
- 2 tablespoons of olive oil
- Black pepper to the taste
- ½ cup of low-sodium veggie stock
- 1 tablespoon of cilantro, chopped

DIRECTIONS

1. Heat a pan with the oil over medium heat, add the scallions and the garlic, toss and cook for 5 minutes.
2. Add the meat, toss and cook for 5 minutes more.
3. Add the rest of the ingredients, bring to a simmer and cook over medium heat for 20 minutes.
4. Divide the mix between plates and serve.

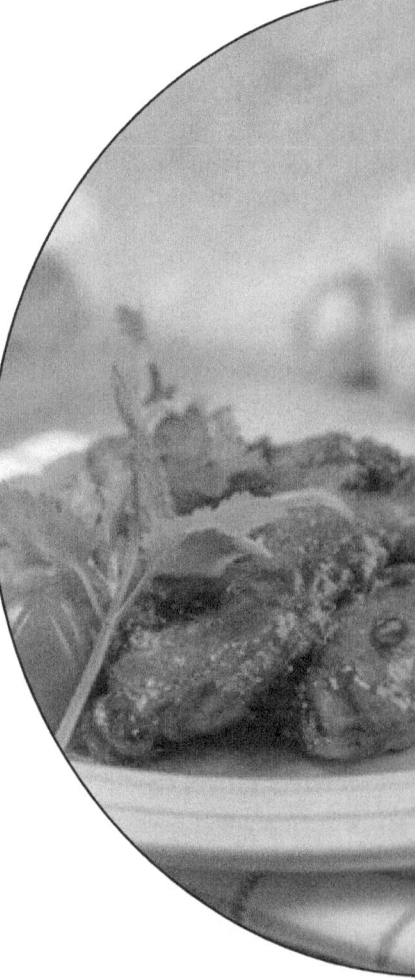

BALSAMIC PORK

Preparation Time: 10 minutes
Cooking Time: 30 minutes
Servings: 2

INGREDIENTS

- 1 red onion, sliced
- 1 pound of pork stew meat, cubed
- 2 red chilies, chopped
- 2 tablespoons of balsamic vinegar
- ½ cup of coriander leaves, chopped
- Black pepper to the taste
- 2 tablespoons of olive oil
- 1 tablespoon of low-sodium tomato sauce

DIRECTIONS

1. Heat a pan with the oil over medium heat, add the onion and the chilies, toss and cook for 5 minutes.
2. Add the meat, toss and cook for 5 minutes more.
3. Add the rest of the ingredients, toss, bring to a simmer and cook over medium heat for 20 minutes more.
4. Divide everything between plates and serve right away.

PESTO PORK

Preparation Time: 10 minutes
Cooking Time: 36 minutes
Servings: 2

INGREDIENTS

- 2 tablespoons of olive oil
- 2 spring onions, chopped
- 1 pound of pork chops
- 2 tablespoons of basil pesto
- 1 cup of cherry tomatoes, cubed
- 2 tablespoons of low-sodium tomato paste
- ½ cup of parsley, chopped
- ½ cup of low-sodium veggie stock
- Black pepper to the taste

DIRECTIONS

1. Heat a pan with the olive oil over medium-high heat, add the spring onions and the pork chops, and brown for 3 minutes on each side.
2. Add the pesto and the other ingredients, toss gently, bring to a simmer and cook over medium heat for 30 minutes more.
3. Divide everything between plates and serve.

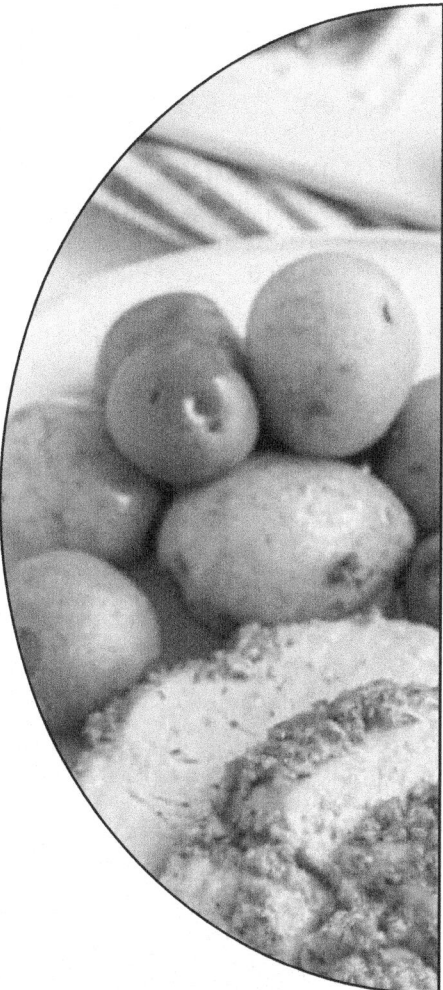

PORK AND PARSLEY PEPPERS

Preparation Time: 10 minutes
Cooking Time: 1 hour
Servings: 2

INGREDIENTS

- 1 green bell pepper, chopped
- 1 red bell pepper, chopped
- 1 yellow bell pepper, chopped
- 1 red onion, chopped
- 1 pound of pork chops
- 1 tablespoon of olive oil
- Black pepper to the taste
- 26 ounces of canned tomatoes, no-salt-added and chopped
- 2 tablespoons of parsley, chopped

DIRECTIONS

1. Grease a roasting pan with the oil, arrange the pork chops inside and add the other ingredients on top.
2. Bake at 390 ºF for 1 hour, divide everything between plates and serve.

CUMIN LAMB MIX

Preparation Time: 10 minutes
Cooking Time: 25 minutes
Servings: 2

INGREDIENTS

- 1 tablespoon of olive oil
- 1 red onion, chopped
- 1 cup of cherry tomatoes, halved
- 1 pound of lamb stew meat, ground
- 1 tablespoon of chili powder
- Black pepper to the taste
- 2 teaspoons of cumin, ground
- 1 cup of low-sodium veggie stock
- 2 tablespoons of cilantro, chopped

DIRECTIONS

1. Heat the pan with the oil over medium-high heat, add the onion, lamb and chili powder, toss and cook for 10 minutes.
2. Add the rest of the ingredients, toss, and cook over medium heat for 15 minutes more.
3. Divide into bowls and serve.

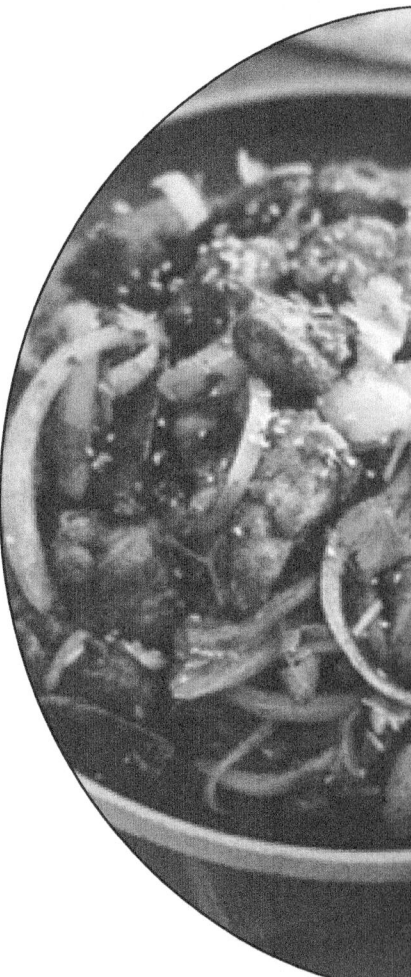

PORK WITH RADISHES AND GREEN BEANS

Preparation Time: 10 minutes
Cooking Time: 35 minutes
Servings: 2

INGREDIENTS

- 1 pound of pork stew meat, cubed
- 1 cup of radishes, cubed
- ½ pound of green beans, trimmed and halved
- 1 yellow onion, chopped
- 1 tablespoon of olive oil
- 2 garlic cloves, minced
- 1 cup of canned tomatoes, no-salt-added and chopped
- 2 teaspoons of oregano, dried
- Black pepper to the taste

DIRECTIONS

1. Heat a pan with the oil over medium-high heat, add the onion and the garlic, toss and cook for 5 minutes.
2. Add the meat, toss and cook for 5 minutes more.
3. Add the rest of the ingredients, bring to a simmer and cook over medium heat for 25 minutes.
4. Divide everything into bowls and serve.

FENNEL LAMB AND MUSHROOMS

Preparation Time: 10 minutes
Cooking Time: 40 minutes
Servings: 2

INGREDIENTS

- 1 pound of lamb shoulder, boneless and cubed
- 8 white mushrooms, halved
- 2 tablespoons of olive oil
- 1 yellow onion, chopped
- 2 garlic cloves, minced
- 1 an ½ tablespoons of fennel powder
- Black pepper to the taste
- A bunch of scallions, chopped
- 1 cup of low-sodium veggie stock

DIRECTIONS

1. Heat a pan with the oil over medium heat, add the onion and the garlic, toss and cook for 5 minutes.
2. Add the meat and the mushrooms, toss and cook for 5 minutes more.
3. Add the other ingredients, toss, bring to a simmer and cook over medium heat for 30 minutes.
4. Divide the mix into bowls and serve.

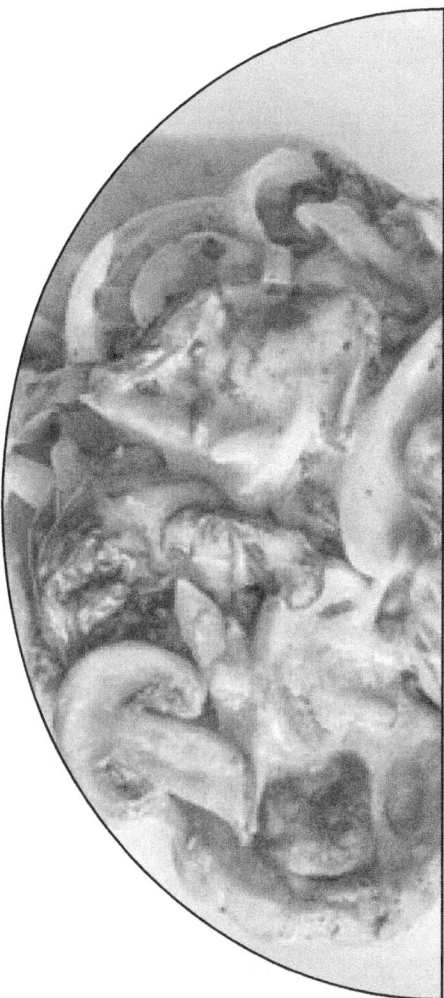

PORK AND SPINACH PAN

Preparation Time: 10 minutes
Cooking Time: 30 minutes
Servings: 2

INGREDIENTS

- 1 pound of pork, ground
- 2 tablespoons of olive oil
- 1 red onion, chopped
- ½ pound of baby spinach
- 4 garlic cloves, minced
- ½ cup of low-sodium veggie stock
- ½ cup of canned tomatoes, no-salt-added, chopped
- Black pepper to the taste
- 1 tablespoon of chives, chopped

DIRECTIONS

1. Heat a pan with the oil over medium-high heat, add the onion and the garlic, toss and cook for 5 minutes.
2. Add the meat, toss and brown for 5 minutes more.
3. Add the rest of the ingredients except the spinach, toss, bring to a simmer, reduce heat to medium and cook for 15 minutes.
4. Add the spinach, toss, cook the mix for another 5 minutes, divide everything into bowls and serve.

PORK WITH AVOCADOS

Preparation Time: 10 minutes
Cooking Time: 15 minutes
Servings: 2

INGREDIENTS

- 2 cups of baby spinach
- 1 pound of pork steak, cut into strips
- 1 tablespoon of olive oil
- 1 cup of cherry tomatoes, halved
- 2 avocados, peeled, pitted and cut into wedges
- 1 tablespoon of balsamic vinegar
- ½ cup of low-sodium veggie stock

DIRECTIONS

1. Heat a pan with the oil over medium-high heat, add the meat, toss and cook for 10 minutes.
2. Add the spinach and the other ingredients, toss, cook for 5 minutes more, divide into bowls and serve.

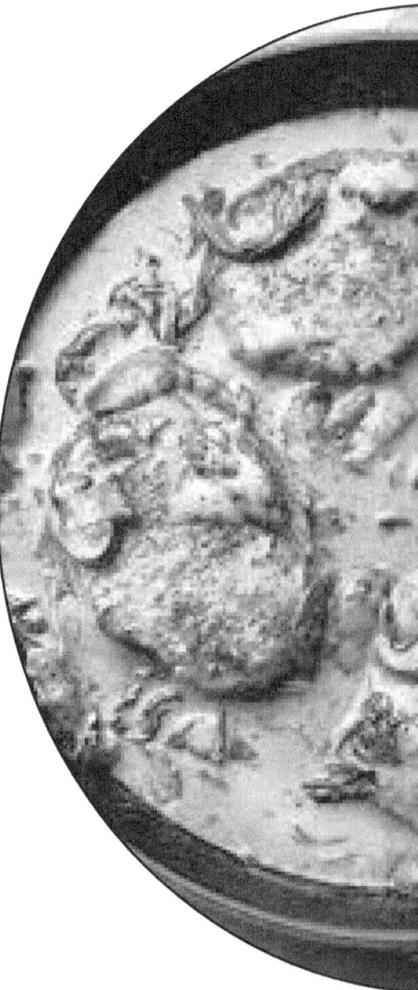

PORK AND SPINACH PAN

Preparation Time: 10 minutes
Cooking Time: 40 minutes
Servings: 2

INGREDIENTS

- 2 pounds of pork stew meat, cut into strips
- 2 green apples, cored and cut into wedges
- 2 garlic cloves, minced
- 2 shallots, chopped
- 1 tablespoon of sweet paprika
- ½ teaspoon of chili powder
- 2 tablespoons of avocado oil
- 1 cup of low-sodium chicken stock
- Black pepper to the taste
- A pinch of red chili pepper flakes

DIRECTIONS

1. Heat a pan with the oil over medium heat; add the shallots and the garlic, toss and sauté for 5 minutes.
2. Add the meat and brown for another 5 minutes.
3. Add the apples and the other ingredients; toss, bring to a simmer and cook over medium heat for 30 minutes more.
4. Divide everything between plates and serve.

CINNAMON PORK CHOPS

Preparation Time: 10 minutes
Cooking Time: 1 hour and 10 minutes
Servings: 2

INGREDIENTS

- 4 pork chops
- 2 tablespoons of olive oil
- 2 garlic cloves, minced
- ¼ cup of low-sodium veggie stock
- 1 tablespoon of cinnamon powder
- Black pepper to the taste
- 1 teaspoon of chili powder
- ½ teaspoon of onion powder

DIRECTIONS

1. In a roasting pan, combine the pork chops with the oil and the other ingredients, toss, introduce in the oven and bake at 390 ° F for 1 hour and 10 minutes.
2. Divide the pork chops between plates and serve with a side salad.

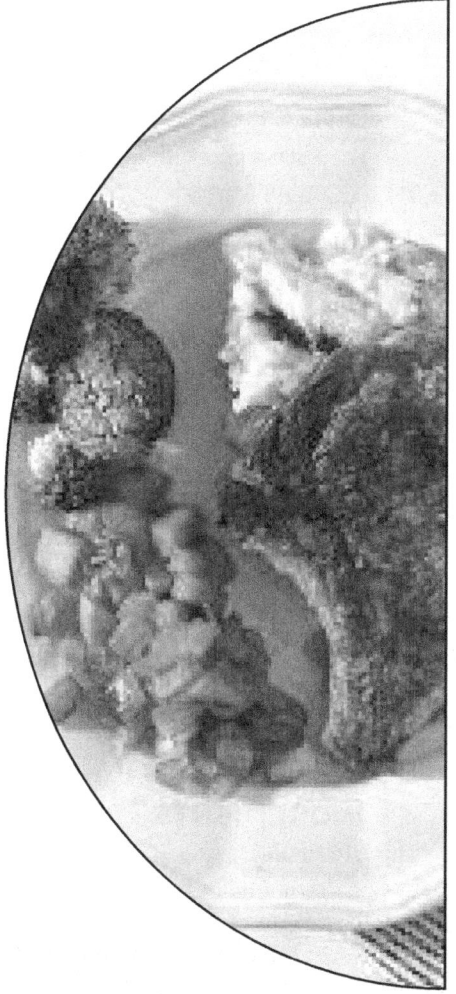

COCONUT PORK CHOPS

Preparation Time: 10 minutes
Cooking Time: 20 minutes
Servings: 2

INGREDIENTS

- 2 tablespoons of olive oil
- 4 pork chops
- 1 yellow onion, chopped
- 1 tablespoon of chili powder
- 1 cup of coconut milk
- ¼ cup of cilantro, chopped

DIRECTIONS

1. Heat a pan with the oil over medium-high heat; add the onion and the chili powder, toss and sauté for 5 minutes.
2. Add the pork chops and brown them for 2 minutes on each side.
3. Add the coconut milk, toss, bring to a simmer and cook over medium heat for 11 minutes more.
4. Add the cilantro, toss, divide everything into bowls and serve.

PORK WITH PEACHES MIX

Preparation Time: 10 minutes
Cooking Time: 25 minutes
Servings: 2

INGREDIENTS

- 2 pounds of pork tenderloin, roughly cubed
- 2 peaches, stones removed and cut into quarters
- ¼ teaspoon of onion powder
- 2 tablespoons of olive oil
- ¼ teaspoon of smoked paprika
- ¼ cup of low-sodium veggie stock
- Black pepper to the taste

DIRECTIONS

1. Heat a pan with the oil over medium heat, add the meat, toss and cook for 10 minutes.
2. Add the peaches and the other ingredients; toss, bring to a simmer and cook over medium heat for 15 minutes more.
3. Divide the whole mix between plates and serve.

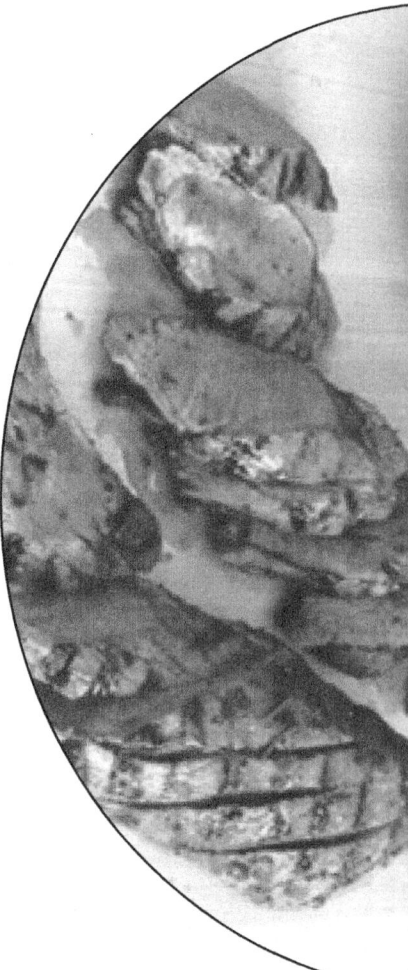

COCOA LAMB AND RADISHES

Preparation Time: 10 minutes
Cooking Time: 35 minutes
Servings: 2

INGREDIENTS

- ½ cup of low-sodium veggie stock
- 1 pound of lamb stew meat, cubed
- 1 cup of radishes, cubed
- 1 tablespoon of cocoa powder
- Black pepper to the taste
- 1 yellow onion, chopped
- 1 tablespoon of olive oil
- 2 garlic cloves, minced
- 1 tablespoon of parsley, chopped

DIRECTIONS

1. Heat a pan with the oil over medium-high heat; add the onion and the garlic, toss and sauté for 5 minutes.
2. Add the meat, toss and brown for 2 minutes on each side.
3. Add the stock and the other ingredients; toss, bring to a simmer and cook over medium heat for 25 minutes more.
4. Divide everything between plates and serve.

BEEF AND SAUERKRAUT SOUP RECIPE

Preparation Time: 35 minutes
Cooking Time: 1 hour 30 minutes
Servings: 2

INGREDIENTS

- 1 pound of beef; ground
- 14 ounces of beef stock
- 2 cups of chicken stock
- 3 teaspoons of olive oil
- 2 cups of water
- 1 tablespoon of gluten-free Worcestershire sauce
- 3 tablespoons of parsley; chopped.
- Salt and black pepper, to the taste.
- 4 bay leaves
- 1 onion; chopped.
- 1 tablespoon of stevia
- 1 teaspoon of sage; dried
- 1 tablespoon of garlic; minced
- 14 ounces of canned tomatoes and juice
- 14 ounces of sauerkraut; chopped.

DIRECTIONS

1. Heat a pan with 1 teaspoon of oil over medium heat; add beef; stir, and brown for 10 minutes.
2. Meanwhile, in a pot, mix chicken and beef stock with sauerkraut, stevia, canned tomatoes, Worcestershire sauce, parsley, sage and bay leaves; stir and bring to a simmer over medium heat.
3. Add the beef to soup; stir, and continue simmering.
4. Heat up the same pan with the rest of the oil over medium heat; add onions; stir and cook for 2 minutes.
5. Add the garlic; stir, cook for 1 minute more and add this to the soup.
6. Reduce heat to soup and simmer it for 1 hour.
7. Add the salt, pepper and water; stir and cook for 15 minutes more
8. Divide into bowls and serve.

NUTRITION

- Calories: 250
- Fat: 5 g
- Fiber: 1 g
- Carbs: 3 g
- Protein: 12 g

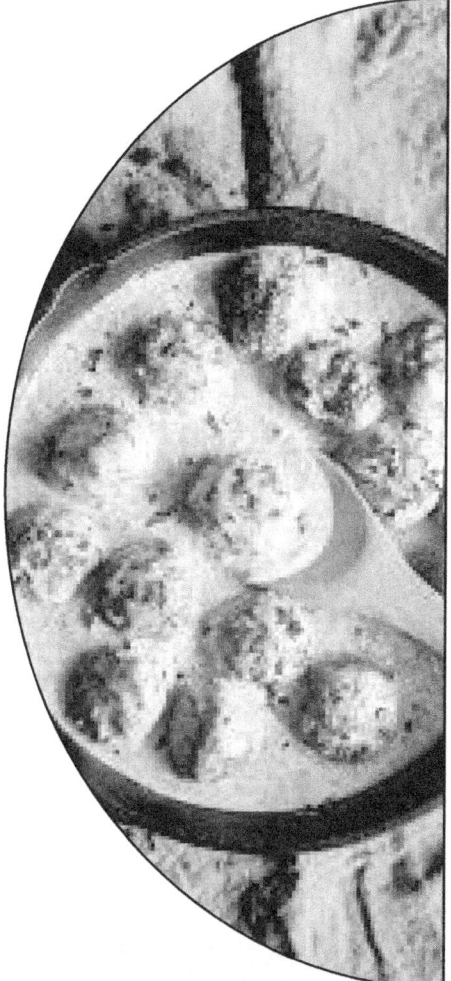

MEATBALLS AND MUSHROOM SAUCE

Preparation Time: 35 minutes
Cooking Time: 15 minutes
Servings: 2

INGREDIENTS

- 2 pounds beef; ground
- 1 tablespoon of coconut aminos
- 1/2 teaspoon of garlic powder
- 1 tablespoon of parsley; chopped.
- 1 tablespoon of onion flakes
- 1/4 cup of beef stock
- ¾ cup of almond flour
- Salt and black pepper to the taste.

- For the sauce:
- 1 cup of yellow onion; chopped.
- 2 cups of mushrooms; sliced
- 1/2 teaspoon of coconut aminos
- 1/4 cup of sour cream
- 1/2 cup of beef stock
- 2 tablespoons of bacon fat
- 2 tablespoons of ghee
- Salt and black pepper to the taste.

DIRECTIONS

1. In a bowl, mix beef with salt, pepper, garlic powder, 1 tablespoon of coconut aminos, 1/4 cup beef stock, almond flour, parsley and onion flakes; stir well, shape 6 patties, place them on a baking sheet, introduce in the oven at 375 ºF and bake for 18 minutes.
2. Meanwhile; heat a pan with the ghee and the bacon fat over medium heat; add mushrooms; stir and cook for 4 minutes.
3. Add the onions; stir, and cook for 4 minutes more.
4. Add 1/2 teaspoon of coconut aminos, sour cream and 1/2 cup beef stock; stir well and bring to a simmer.
5. Take off heat; add salt and pepper, and stir well.
6. Divide beef patties between plates and serve with mushroom sauce on top.

NUTRITION

- Calories: 435
- Fat: 23 g
- Fiber: 4 g
- Carbs: 6 g
- Protein: 32 g

LAMB CASSEROLE

Preparation Time: 35 minutes
Cooking Time: 1 hour 50 minutes
Servings: 2

INGREDIENTS

- 2 carrots; chopped.
- 1/2 tablespoon of rosemary; chopped.
- 1/2 cauliflower; florets separated
- 1/2 celeriac; chopped.
- 2 garlic cloves; minced
- 1¼ cups of lamb stock
- 1 red onion; chopped.
- 1 leek; chopped.
- 1 tablespoon of olive oil
- 1 celery stick; chopped.
- 1 tablespoon of mint sauce
- 1 teaspoon of stevia
- 1 tablespoon of tomato puree
- 2 tablespoons of ghee
- 10 ounces of lamb fillet; cut into medium pieces
- Salt and black pepper to the taste.

DIRECTIONS

1. Heat a pot with the oil over medium heat; add garlic, onion and celery; stir and cook for 5 minutes.
2. Add the lamb pieces; stir and cook for 3 minutes.
3. Add the carrot, leek, rosemary, stock, tomato puree, mint sauce and stevia; stir, bring to a boil, cover and cook for 1 hour and 30 minutes.
4. Heat a pot with water over medium heat; add celeriac, cover and simmer for 10 minutes.
5. Add the cauliflower florets, cook for 15 minutes, drain everything and mix with salt, pepper and ghee.
6. Mash using a potato masher and divide mash between plates.
7. Add the lamb and veggies mix on top and serve.

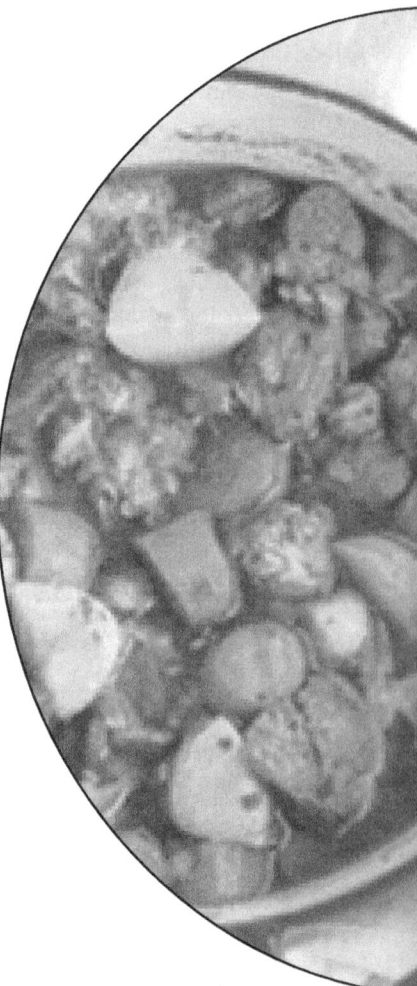

THAI BEEF RECIPE

Preparation Time: 20 minutes
Cooking Time: 15 minutes
Servings: 2

INGREDIENTS

- 1 pound of beef steak; cut into strips
- 1 cup of beef stock
- 1½ teaspoons of lemon pepper
- 4 tablespoons of peanut butter
- 1/4 teaspoon of garlic powder
- 1/4 teaspoon of onion powder
- 1 tablespoon of coconut aminos
- 1 green bell pepper; chopped.
- 3 green onions; chopped.
- Salt and black pepper, to the taste.

DIRECTIONS

1. In a bowl, mix peanut butter with stock, aminos and lemon pepper; stir well and leave aside.
2. Heat a pan over medium-high heat; add beef, season with salt, pepper, onion and garlic powder and cook for 7 minutes.
3. Add green pepper; stir, and cook for 3 minutes more.
4. Add peanut sauce you've made at the beginning and green onions; stir, cook for 1 minute more, divide between plates and serve.

GOULASH

Preparation Time: 30 minutes
Cooking Time: 15 minutes
Servings: 2

INGREDIENTS

- 2 ounces of bell pepper; chopped.
- 2 cups of cauliflower florets
- 1/4 teaspoon of garlic powder
- 1½ pounds of beef; ground
- 14 ounces of canned tomatoes and their juice
- 1 tablespoon of tomato paste
- 14 ounces of water
- 1/4 cup of onion; chopped
- Salt and black pepper, to the taste

DIRECTIONS

1. Heat a pan over medium heat; add beef; stir and brown for 5 minutes.
2. Add the onion and bell pepper; stir and cook for 4 minutes more.
3. Add the cauliflower, tomatoes and their juice and water; stir, bring to a simmer, cover pan and cook for 5 minutes.
4. Add the tomato paste, garlic powder, salt and pepper; stir, take off heat; divide into bowls and serve.

NUTRITION

- Calories: 275
- Fat: 7 g
- Fiber: 2 g
- Carbs: 4 g
- Protein: 10 g

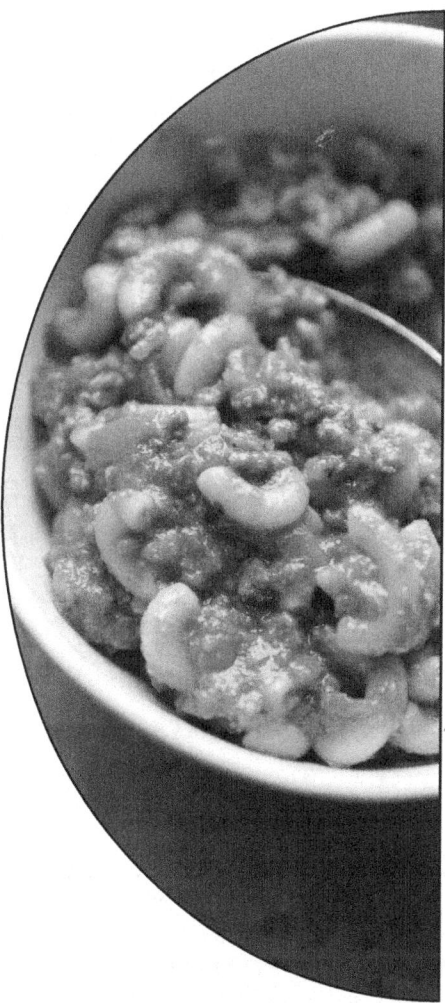

LAMB AND MUSTARD SAUCE

Preparation Time: 30 minutes
Cooking Time: 20 minutes
Servings: 2

INGREDIENTS

- 2/3 cup of heavy cream
- 1/2 cup of beef stock
- 1 tablespoon of mustard
- 2 teaspoons of gluten-free Worcestershire sauce
- 1½ pounds of lamb chops
- 2 tablespoons of olive oil
- 1 tablespoon of fresh rosemary; chopped
- 2 garlic cloves; minced
- 1 teaspoon of Erythritol
- 2 tablespoons of ghee
- A spring of rosemary
- A spring of thyme
- 1 tablespoon of shallot; chopped.
- 2 teaspoons of lemon juice
- Salt and black pepper to the taste

DIRECTIONS

1. In a bowl, mix 1 tablespoon of oil with garlic, salt, pepper and rosemary and whisk well.
2. Add the lamb chops, toss to coat and leave aside for a few minutes.
3. Heat a pan with the rest of the oil over medium-high heat; add lamb chops, reduce heat to medium, cook them for 7 minutes, flip, cook them for 7 minutes more, transfer to a plate and keep them warm.
4. Return the pan to medium heat; add shallots; stir, and cook for 3 minutes.
5. Add the stock; stir, and cook for 1 minute.
6. Add the Worcestershire sauce, mustard, Erythritol, cream, rosemary and thyme spring; stir and cook for 8 minutes.
7. Add the lemon juice, salt, pepper and ghee, discard rosemary and thyme; stir well and take off the heat.
8. Divide the lamb chops on plates, drizzle the sauce over them and serve.

NUTRITION

- Calories: 435
- Fat: 30 g
- Fiber: 4 g
- Carbs: 5 g
- Protein: 32 g

BEEF ZUCCHINI CUPS

Preparation Time: 45 minutes
Cooking Time: 30 minutes
Servings: 2

INGREDIENTS

- 1 pound of beef; ground
- 2 garlic cloves; minced
- 1 teaspoon of cumin; ground
- 1 tablespoon of coconut oil
- 1/2 cup of red onion; chopped.
- 1/2 cup of cheddar cheese; shredded
- 1½ cups of enchilada sauce
- 1 teaspoon of smoked paprika
- 3 zucchinis; sliced in halves length-wise and insides scooped out
- 1/4 cup of cilantro; chopped
- Some chopped avocado for serving
- Some green onions; chopped for serving
- Some tomatoes; chopped for serving
- Salt and black pepper to the taste.

DIRECTIONS

1. Heat a pan with the oil over medium-high heat; add red onions; stir, and cook for 2 minutes.
2. Add the beef, stir and brown for a couple of minutes.
3. Add the paprika, salt, pepper, cumin and garlic; stir and cook for 2 minutes.
4. Place the zucchini halves in a baking pan, stuff each with beef, pour enchilada sauce on top and sprinkle cheddar cheese.
5. Bake covered in the oven at 350 ºF for 20 minutes.
6. Uncover the pan, sprinkle cilantro and bake for 5 minutes more.
7. Sprinkle avocado, green onions and tomatoes on top, divide between plates and serve.

NUTRITION

- Calories: 222
- Fat: 10 g
- Fiber: 2 g
- Carbs: 8 g
- Protein: 21 g

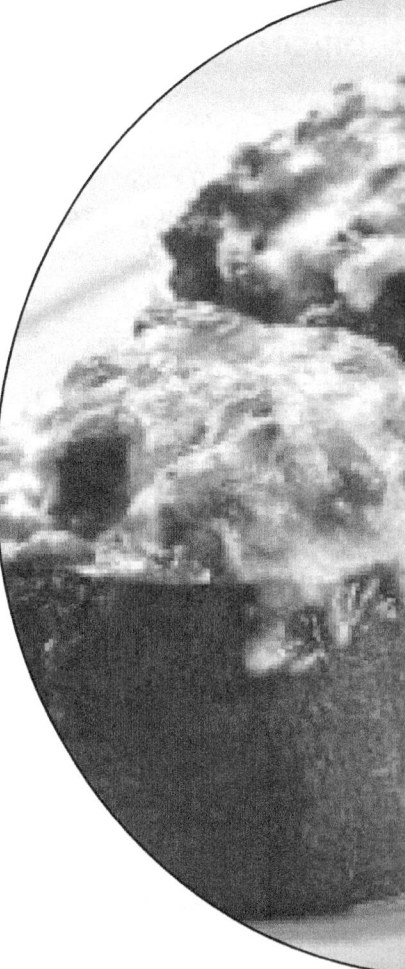

BEEF AND TZATZIKI

Preparation Time: 25 minutes
Cooking Time: 15 minutes
Servings: 2

INGREDIENTS

- 17 ounces of beef; ground
- 7 ounces of cherry tomatoes; cut in halves
- 1/4 cup of almond milk
- 1 yellow onion; grated
- 5 bread slices; torn
- 1 egg; whisked
- 1/4 cup of olive oil
- 1 cucumber; thinly sliced
- 1 cup of baby spinach 1/4 cup of parsley; chopped
- 2 garlic of cloves; minced
- 1/4 cup of mint; chopped
- 2½ teaspoons of oregano; dried
- 7 ounces of jarred Tzatziki
- Salt and black pepper to the taste

DIRECTIONS

1. Put the torn bread in a bowl, add milk and leave aside for 3 minutes.
2. Squeeze bread, chop and put into a bowl.
3. Add the beef, egg, salt, pepper, oregano, mint, parsley, garlic and onion and stir well.
4. Shape balls from this mix and place them on a working surface.
5. Heat a pan with half of the oil over medium-high heat; add meatballs, cook them for 8 minutes, flipping them from time to time and transfer them all to a tray.
6. In a salad bowl, mix spinach with cucumber and tomato.
7. Add the meatballs, the rest of the oil, some salt, pepper and lemon juice.
8. Also, add the Tzatziki, toss to coat and serve.

NUTRITION

- Calories: 200
- Fat: 4 g
- Fiber: 1 g
- Carbs: 3 g
- Protein: 7 g

BEEF AND TOMATO STUFFED SQUASH

Preparation Time: 1 hour 10 minutes
Cooking Time: 10 minutes
Servings: 2

INGREDIENTS

- 28 ounces of canned tomatoes; chopped.
- 2 pounds of spaghetti squash; pricked with a fork
- 1/2 teaspoon of thyme; dried
- 1 pound of beef; ground
- 1 green bell pepper; chopped.
- 3 garlic cloves; minced
- 1 yellow onion; chopped.
- 1 Portobello mushroom; sliced
- 1 teaspoon of oregano; dried
- 1/4 teaspoon of cayenne pepper
- Salt and black pepper to the taste

DIRECTIONS

1. Place the spaghetti squash on a lined baking sheet, introduce in the oven at 400 °F and bake for 40 minutes.
2. Cut in half, leave aside to cool down, remove seeds and leave aside.
3. Heat a pan over medium-high heat; add meat, garlic, onion and mushroom; stir and cook until meat browns.
4. Add the salt, pepper, thyme, oregano, cayenne, tomatoes and green pepper; stir and cook for 10 minutes.
5. Stuff squash halves with this beef mix, introduce in the oven at 400 °F and bake for 10 minutes.
6. Divide between 2 plates and serve.

NUTRITION

- Calories: 260
- Fat: 7 g
- Fiber: 2 g
- Carbs: 4 g
- Protein: 10 g

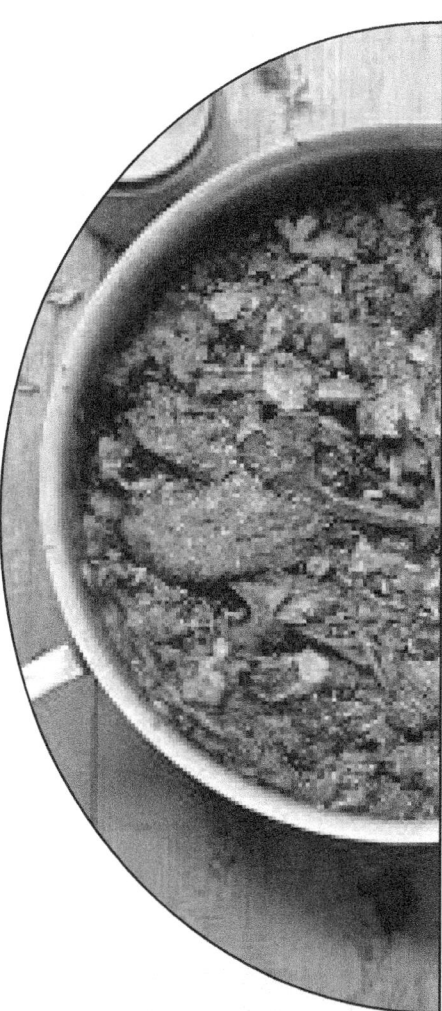

BRAISED LAMB CHOPS

Preparation Time: 10 minutes
Cooking Time: 2 hours 40 minutes
Servings: 2

INGREDIENTS

- 1 teaspoon of garlic powder
- 1 shallot; chopped
- 1 cup of white wine
- 1 bay leaf
- 2 cups of beef stock
- 8 lamb chops
- Some chopped parsley for serving
- 2 teaspoons of mint; crushed
- A drizzle of olive oil
- Juice of 1/2 lemon
- Salt and black pepper to the taste

For the sauce:
- 2 cups of cranberries
- 1/2 teaspoon of rosemary; chopped.
- 1 teaspoon of ginger; grated
- 1 cup of water
- 1/2 cup of swerve
- 1 teaspoon of mint; dried
- Juice of 1/2 lemon
- 1 teaspoon of harass paste

DIRECTIONS

1. In a bowl, mix lamb chops with salt, pepper, 1 teaspoon of garlic powder and 2 teaspoons of mint and rub well.
2. Heat a pan with a drizzle of oil over medium-high heat; add lamb chops, brown them on all sides and transfer to a plate.
3. Heat the same pan again over medium-high heat; add shallots; stir, and cook for 1 minute.
4. Add the wine and bay leaf; stir and cook for 4 minutes.
5. Add 2 cups beef stock, parsley and juice from 1/2 lemon; stir and simmer for 5 minutes.
6. Return the lamb; stir, and cook for 10 minutes.
7. Cover the pan and introduce it in the oven at 350 °F for 2 hours.
8. Meanwhile; heat a pan over medium-high heat; add cranberries, swerve, rosemary, 1 teaspoon of mint, juice from 1/2 lemon, ginger, water and harissa paste; stir, bring to a simmer for 15 minutes.
9. Take the lamb chops out of the oven, divide them between plates, drizzle the cranberry sauce over them and serve.

NUTRITION

- Calories: 450
- Fat: 34 g
- Fiber: 2 g
- Carbs: 6 g
- Protein: 26 g

LAMB WITH FENNEL

Preparation Time: 50 minutes
Cooking Time: 40 minutes
Servings: 2

INGREDIENTS

- 12 ounces of lamb racks
- 1 tablespoon of swerve
- 4 figs; cut in halves
- 2 fennel bulbs; sliced
- 2 tablespoons of olive oil
- 1/8 cup of apple cider vinegar
- Salt and black pepper to the taste

DIRECTIONS

1. In a bowl, mix the fennel with figs, vinegar, swerve and oil, toss to coat well and transfer to a baking dish.
2. Season with salt and pepper, introduce in the oven at 400 °F and bake for 15 minutes.
3. Season the lamb with salt and pepper, place into a heated pan over medium-high heat and cook for a couple of minutes.
4. Add the lamb to the baking dish with the fennel and figs, introduce in the oven and bake for 20 more minutes.
5. Divide everything between plates and serve.

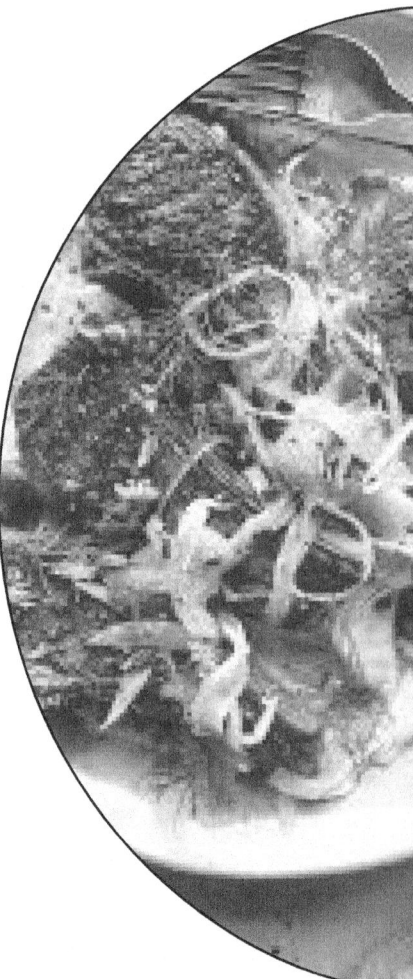

BEEF AND EGGPLANT CASSEROLE

Preparation Time: 10 minutes
Cooking Time: 4 hours 30 minutes
Servings: 2

INGREDIENTS

- 2 pounds of beef; ground
- 2 cups of mozzarella; grated
- 1 tablespoon of olive oil
- 2 cups of eggplant; chopped
- 16 ounces of tomato sauce
- 1 teaspoon of oregano; dried
- 2 teaspoons of mustard
- 2 tablespoons of parsley; chopped
- 2 teaspoons of gluten-free Worcestershire sauce
- 28 ounces of canned tomatoes; chopped
- Salt and black pepper, to the taste

DIRECTIONS

1. Season the eggplant pieces with salt and pepper, leave them aside for 30 minutes, squeeze water a bit, put them into a bowl, add the olive oil and toss them to coat.
2. In another bowl, mix the beef with salt, pepper, mustard, and Worcestershire sauce. Stir well.
3. Press them on the bottom of a crock-pot.
4. Add the eggplant and spread.
5. Also, add tomatoes, tomato sauce, parsley, oregano and mozzarella.
6. Cover the Crockpot and cook on Low for 4 hours.
7. Divide casserole between plates and serve hot.

BURGUNDY BEEF STEW RECIPE

Preparation Time: 30 minutes
Cooking Time: 3 hours 10 minutes
Servings: 2

INGREDIENTS

- 15 ounces of canned tomatoes; chopped
- 2 yellow onions; chopped
- 3 tablespoons of almond flour
- 1 cup of water
- 4 carrots; chopped
- 1 cup of beef stock
- 1 tablespoon of thyme; chopped
- 1/2 teaspoon of mustard powder
- 1/2 pounds of mushrooms; sliced
- 2 celery ribs; chopped
- Salt and black pepper, to the taste

DIRECTIONS

1. Heat an oven proof pot over medium-high heat; add beef cubes; stir and brown them for a couple of minutes on each side.
2. Add the tomatoes, mushrooms, onions, carrots, celery, salt, pepper mustard, stock, thyme and stir.
3. In a bowl, mix water with flour and stir well.
4. Add this to the pot; stir well, introduce in the oven and bake at 325 ºF for 3 hours.
5. Stir every half an hour. Divide into bowls and serve.

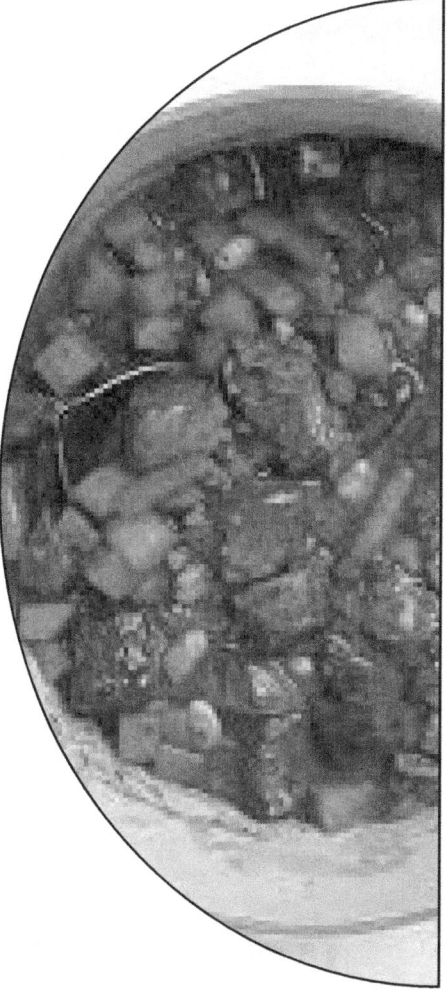

BEEF ROAST

Preparation Time: 20 minutes
Cooking Time: 1 hour 25 minutes
Servings: 2

INGREDIENTS
- 3½ pounds of beef roast
- 1-ounce of onion soup mix
- 1/2 cup of Italian dressing
- 12 ounces of beef stock
- 4 ounces of mushrooms; sliced

DIRECTIONS
1. In a bowl, mix the stock with onion soup mix and Italian dressing and stir.
2. Put beef roast in a pan, add mushrooms, stock mix, cover with tin foil, introduce in the oven at 300 ºF and bake for 1 hour and 15 minutes.
3. Leave roast to cool down a bit, slice and serve with the gravy on top.

LAMB

Preparation Time: 10 minutes
Cooking Time: 8 hours 10 minutes
Servings: 2

INGREDIENTS

- 2 pounds of lamb leg
- 6 mint leaves
- 1 tablespoon of maple extract
- 2 tablespoons of mustard
- 1/4 cup of olive oil
- 1 teaspoon of garlic; minced
- A pinch of rosemary; dried
- 4 thyme spring
- Salt and black pepper, to the taste

DIRECTIONS

1. Put the oil in your slow cooker.
2. Add the lamb, salt, pepper, maple extract, mustard, rosemary and garlic, rub well, cover and cook on Low for 7 hours.
3. Add the mint and thyme and cook for 1 more hour.
4. Leave the lamb to cool down a bit before slicing and serving with pan juices on top.

NUTRITION

- Calories: 400
- Fat: 34 g
- Fiber: 1 g
- Carbs: 3 g
- Protein: 26 g

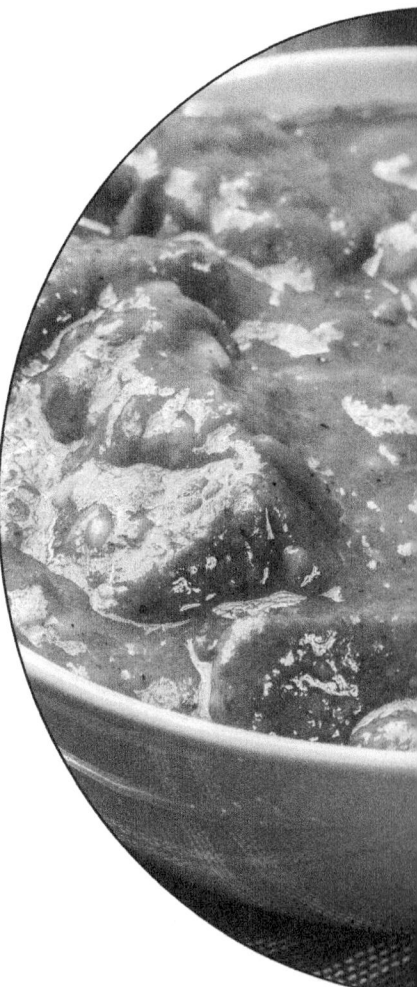

CHAPTER 6.
SALADS & SOUPS

EASY SHRIMP SALAD

Preparation Time: 10 minutes
Cooking Time: 5 minutes
Servings: 2

INGREDIENTS

For the shrimp:
- 2 minced garlic cloves
- 1 lb. of shrimp
- 1 teaspoon of Cajun spice
- 2 tablespoon of olive oil

For the salad:
- 6 c. of lettuce leaves
- 4 chopped tomatoes
- 1 chopped yellow onion
- 1 sliced cucumber
- 2 chopped avocados
- 1 c. of corn
- 1 lemon
- ½ bunch of chopped parsley
- 2 tablespoon of olive oil
- Black pepper

DIRECTIONS

1. In a bowl, combine the shrimp with Cajun spice and garlic and toss.
2. Heat a pan with 2 tablespoons of oil over medium-high heat, add shrimp, cook each side for 2 minutes and set to a bowl.
3. Add the lettuce, tomatoes, onion, cucumber, avocado, corn and a pinch of pepper and toss.
4. In a small bowl, mix 2 tablespoons of oil with parsley and lemon juice, whisk well, pour over the salad, toss and serve for lunch.

NUTRITION
- Calories: 210
- Fat: 4 g
- Carbs: 28 g
- Protein: 14 g

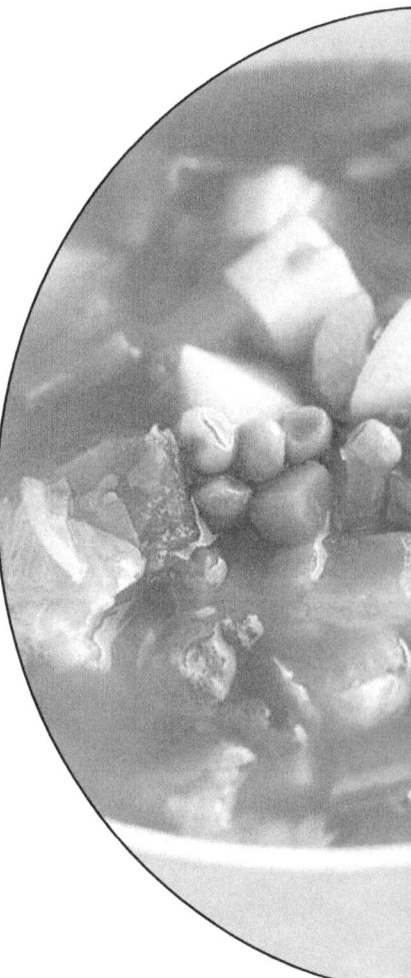

EASY VEGGIE SOUP

Preparation Time: 10 minutes
Cooking Time: 20 minutes
Servings: 2

INGREDIENTS

- 1 tablespoon of olive oil
- 1 chopped yellow onion
- 2 chopped celery ribs
- 2 chopped carrots
- 2 c. of mixed zucchini and cauliflower florets
- black pepper
- 1 teaspoon of dried thyme
- ½ teaspoon of garlic powder
- 1 teaspoon of dried oregano
- 8 c. of veggie stock
- 1 bay leaf
- 14 oz. of chopped canned tomatoes

DIRECTIONS

1. Add the oil in a pot and heat over medium-high heat; add onion, celery and carrots, stir and sauté them for 4 minutes.
2. Add the zucchini, cauliflower, black pepper, thyme, garlic powder, oregano, bay leaf, tomatoes and stock, stir, bring to a simmer and cook for 16 minutes.
3. Stir the soup one more time, ladle it into bowls and serve for a dash diet lunch. Enjoy!

NUTRITION
- Calories: 180
- Fat: 2 g
- Carbs: 28 g
- Protein: 8 g

SEAFOOD SALAD

Preparation Time: 15 minutes
Cooking Time: 1 hour, 40 minutes
Servings: 2

INGREDIENTS

- 1 big octopus
- 1 lb. of mussels
- 2 lbs. of clams
- 1 big squid
- 3 chopped garlic cloves
- 1 celery rib
- ½ c. of sliced celery rib
- 1 carrot
- 1 chopped white onion
- 1 bay leaf
- ¾ c. of veggie stock
- 2 c. of sliced radicchio
- 1 sliced red onion
- 1 c. of chopped parsley
- 1 c. of olive oil
- 1 c. of red wine vinegar
- Black pepper

DIRECTIONS

1. Place the octopus in a large pot with celery rib cut into thirds, garlic, carrot, bay leaf, white onion and stock. Add water to cover the octopus, cover the pot, bring to a boil over high heat, and reduce temperature to low; simmer for 1 hour and 30 minutes. Drain the octopus, reserve boiling liquid and leave it aside to cool down.
2. Put ¼ cup of octopus cooking liquid in another pot, add mussels. Heat up over medium-high heat, cook until they open, transfer to a bowl and leave aside.
3. Add the clams to the pan, cover, cook over medium-high heat until they open as well, transfer to the bowl with mussels and leave aside.
4. Add the squid to the pan, cover and cook over medium-high heat for 3 minutes, transfer to the bowl with mussels and clams.
5. Meanwhile, slice octopus into small pieces and mix with the rest of the seafood.
6. Add the sliced celery, radicchio, red onion, vinegar, olive oil, parsley, salt and pepper, toss and leave aside in the fridge for 2 hours before serving. Enjoy!

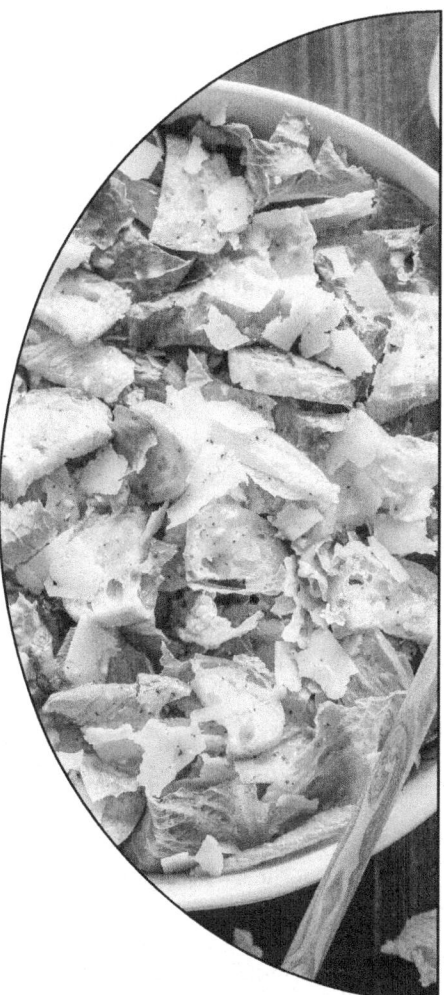

CAESAR SALAD

Preparation Time: 10 minutes
Cooking Time: 10 minutes
Servings: 2

INGREDIENTS

- Cooking spray
- Black pepper
- ½ c. of cubed feta cheese
- 2 tablespoons of lemon juice
- 1½ tablespoon of Dijon mustard
- 1 tablespoon of olive oil
- 1½ tablespoon of red wine vinegar
- ¾ teaspoon of minced garlic
- 1 tablespoon of water
- 1 teaspoon of Worcestershire sauce
- 8 c. of lettuce leaves
- 4 tablespoons of grated parmesan
- 1¼ whole wheat croutons

DIRECTIONS

1. Spray the chicken breasts with some cooking spray and season black pepper to the taste.
2. Heat your kitchen grill over medium-high heat, add chicken breasts, cook for 6 minutes on each side, transfer to a cutting board, cool down for a few minutes, cut in small pieces, transfer to a salad bowl, add lettuce and croutons and leave aside.
3. In your blender, mix feta with lemon juice, olive oil, mustard, vinegar, Worcestershire sauce and garlic and pulse well.
4. Add the water and half of the parmesan and blend some more.
5. Add this to your salad, toss to coat, sprinkle the rest of the parmesan and serve.

GREEK CHICKEN SALAD

Preparation Time: 10 minutes
Cooking Time: 0 minutes
Servings: 2

INGREDIENTS

- 15 oz. of canned chickpeas
- 9 oz. of chicken breast
- 1 chopped cucumber
- 4 chopped green onions
- Salt and Black pepper, to taste
- ½ c. of yogurt
- ¼ c. of chopped mint
- 2 c. of baby spinach
- 2 minced garlic cloves
- 1/3 c. of feta cheese
- 4 lemon wedges

DIRECTIONS

1. In a salad bowl, mix chicken meat with chickpeas, cucumber, onions, mint, garlic, salt and pepper.
2. Add the yogurt, spinach and feta and toss to coat.
3. Serve with lemon wedges on the side.
4. Enjoy!

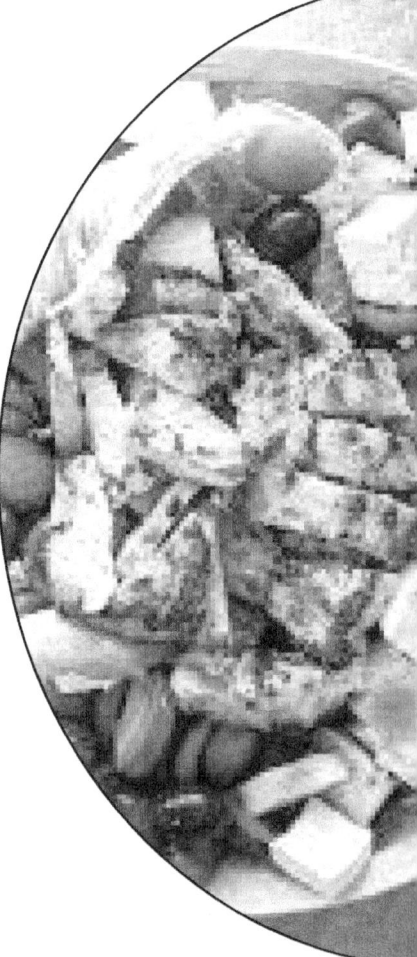

CHICKEN SOUP

Preparation Time: 10 minutes
Cooking Time: 1 hour, 45 minutes
Servings: 2

INGREDIENTS

- 1 whole chicken
- 6 chopped celery stalks
- 6 sliced carrots
- 1 onion
- 1 bunch of parsley springs
- 1 bunch of dill springs
- 2 tablespoons of chopped dill
- 3 garlic cloves
- 2 tablespoons of black peppercorns
- Black pepper
- 2 bay leaves
- ¼ teaspoon of saffron threads

DIRECTIONS

1. Put the chicken pieces in a pot, add water to cover, bring to a boil over medium-high heat, cook for 15 minutes and skim foam.
2. Add the celery, onion, carrots, parsley springs, dill springs, whole garlic cloves, bay leaves, peppercorns, and some black pepper; stir, cover the pot, and reduce heat medium-low and simmer for 1 hour and 30 minutes.
3. Take the chicken pieces out and leave them aside to cool down.
4. Strain soup into another pot, reserve carrots and celery, but discard herbs and spices.
5. Discard bones from the chicken, cut meat into strips and return to pot.
6. Heat the soup with reserved veggies, add chicken pieces, crushed saffron and chopped dill and stir.
7. Ladle the soup into bowls and serve. Enjoy!

PUMPKIN SOUP

Preparation Time: 10 minutes
Cooking Time: 10 minutes
Servings: 2

INGREDIENTS

- 1 chopped yellow onion
- ¾ c. of water
- 15 oz. of pumpkin puree
- 2 c. of veggie stock
- ½ teaspoon of cinnamon powder
- ¼ teaspoon of ground nutmeg
- 1 c. of fat-free milk
- Black pepper
- 1 chopped green onion

DIRECTIONS

1. Put the water in a pot, bring to a simmer over medium heat, add onion, stock, pumpkin puree, and stir.
2. Add the cinnamon, nutmeg, milk and black pepper, stir, cook for 10 minutes, ladle into bowls, sprinkle green onion on top and serve.
3. Enjoy!

NUTRITION

- Calories: 180
- Fat: 10 g
- Carbs: 22 g
- Protein: 14 g

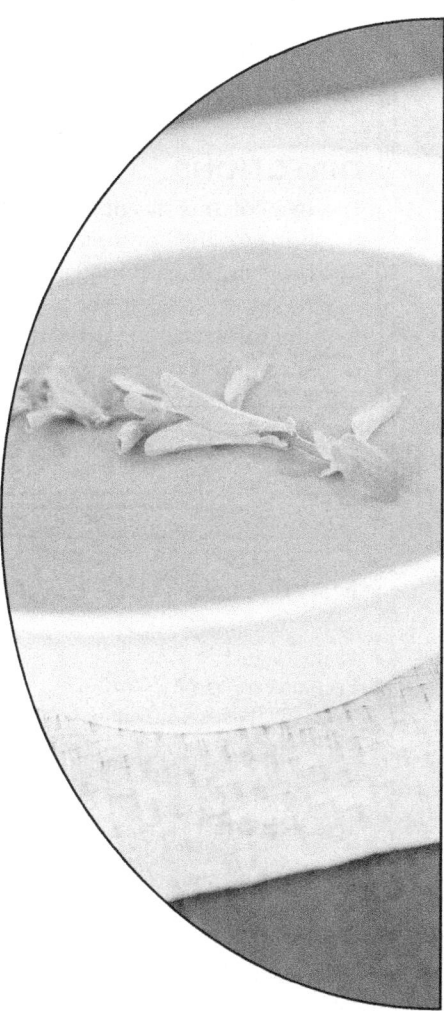

SPICY BLACK BEAN SOUP

Preparation Time: 10 minutes
Cooking Time: 1 hour, 15 minutes
Servings: 2

INGREDIENTS

- 1 lb. of black beans
- 2 chopped yellow onions
- 2 quarts low-sodium veggie stock
- 2 tablespoons of olive oil
- 6 minced garlic cloves
- 2 chopped tomatoes
- 2 chopped jalapenos
- ½ teaspoon of dried oregano
- 1 teaspoon of ground cumin
- 1 teaspoon of grated ginger
- 2 bay leaves
- 1 tablespoon of chili powder
- 3 tablespoon of balsamic vinegar
- Black pepper
- ½ c. of chopped scallions

DIRECTIONS

1. Put the stock in a pot, bring to a simmer over medium heat, add beans, cover and cook for 45 minutes.
2. Meanwhile, heat a pan with the oil over medium-high heat, add ginger, garlic and onion, stir and cook for 5 minutes.
3. Add the tomatoes, cumin, jalapeno, oregano and chili powder, stir, cook for 3 minutes more and transfer to the pot with the beans.
4. Add the bay leaves, and cook the soup for 40 minutes more while the pot is covered.
5. Add the vinegar, stir, cook the soup for 15 minutes more, discard bay leaves, blend the soup using an immersion blender, ladle into bowls and serve with scallions on top. Enjoy!

NUTRITION

- Calories: 220
- Fat: 10 g
- Carbs: 34 g
- Protein: 14 g

SHRIMP SOUP

Preparation Time: 10 minutes
Cooking Time: 25 minutes
Servings: 2

INGREDIENTS

- 8 oz. of shrimp
- 1 stalk lemongrass
- 2 grated ginger
- 6 c. of low-sodium chicken stock
- 2 chopped jalapenos
- 4 lime leaves
- 1½ c. of chopped pineapple
- 1 c. of chopped shiitake mushroom caps
- 1 chopped tomato
- ½ cubed bell pepper
- 1 teaspoon of stevia
- ¼ c. of lime juice
- 1/3 c. of chopped cilantro
- 2 sliced scallions
- 1 tbsp. fish sauce

DIRECTIONS

1. In a pot, mix the ginger with lemongrass, stock, jalapenos and lime leaves, stir, bring to a boil over medium heat, cover, cook for 15 minutes, strain liquid in a bowl and discard solids.
2. Return the soup to the pot, add pineapple, tomato, mushrooms, bell pepper, sugar and fish sauce, stir, bring to a boil over medium heat, cook for 5 minutes, add shrimp and cook for 3 more minutes.
3. Add the lime juice, cilantro and scallions, stir, ladle into soup bowls and serve.
4. Enjoy!

NUTRITION
- Calories: 190
- Fat: 8 g
- Carbs: 30 g
- Protein: 6 g

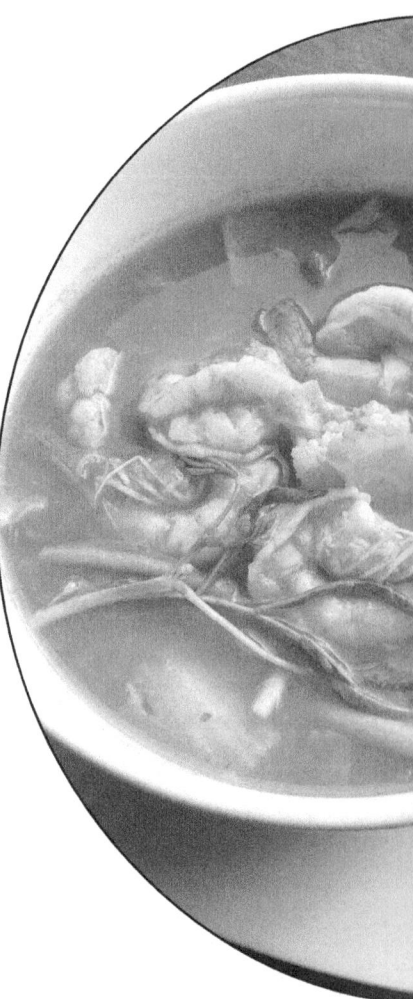

MAYO-LESS TUNA SALAD

Preparation Time: 5 minutes
Cooking Time: 5 minutes
Servings: 2

INGREDIENTS

- 5 oz. of tuna
- 1 tablespoon of extra virgin olive oil
- 1 tablespoon of red wine vinegar
- ¼ c. of chopped green onion
- 2 c. of arugula
- 1 c. of cooked pasta
- 1 tablespoon of Parmesan cheese
- Black pepper

DIRECTIONS

1. Combine all your ingredients into a medium bowl.
2. Split the mixture between two plates.
3. Serve, and enjoy.

NUTRITION
- Calories: 213.2
- Protein: 22.7 g
- Carbs: 20.3 g
- Fat: 6.2 g

CHESTNUT SOUP

Preparation Time: 10 minutes
Cooking Time: 40 minutes
Servings: 2

INGREDIENTS

- 30 oz. of whole roasted chestnuts
- 1 chopped shallot
- ½ c. of heavy cream
- ½ c. of chicken stock
- 1 chopped leek
- ¼ cup of chopped carrots
- 2 tablespoon of butter
- 1 sprig thyme
- 1 bay leaf
- 1 chopped celery stalk
- ½ teaspoon of nutmeg
- Salt
- Pepper

DIRECTIONS

1. Add the butter, carrot, leek, shallot, and celery in a saucepan over medium heat. Cook for 6-7 minutes or until the vegetables are tender.
2. Add the stock, thyme, bay leaf, chestnuts and bring to boil. Reduce heat and simmer for 25 minutes.
3. Remove from the heat and discard the thyme and bay leaf.
4. Allow to cool slightly and puree using an immersion blender.
5. Heat the soup again as you stir in the cream, nutmeg and season to taste.
6. Cook for 5 minutes more.
7. Serve while still hot.

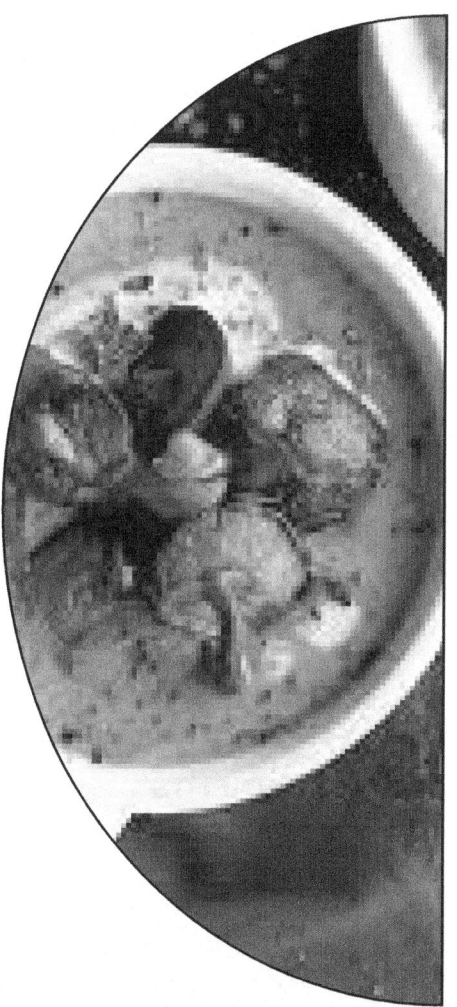

PEPPER POT SOUP

Preparation Time: 10 minutes
Cooking Time: 5 minutes
Servings: 2

INGREDIENTS

- 4 quarts of chicken stock
- 2 diced potatoes
- ½ diced breadfruit
- 1 lb. of diced yam
- ½ lb. of diced cocoa
- 2 crushed garlic cloves
- 2 sprigs of thyme
- 3 chopped green onion
- ½ c. of Coconut Milk
- 10 pimento berries
- 2 chopped callaloo

DIRECTIONS

1. In a reasonable size soup pot, boil 4 quarts of stock.
2. Add garlic, potato, breadfruit, yam, cocoa, and stir.
3. Bring soup to a boil; add thyme, green onion, pimento, callaloo, coconut milk, and pepper.
4. Stir, and cook until done.

QUINOA & AVOCADO SALAD

Preparation Time: 10 minutes
Cooking Time: 5 minutes
Servings: 2

INGREDIENTS

- 1½ c. of cooked quinoa
- 4 oz. of julienned cucumber
- 4 oz. of julienned carrots
- ½ diced avocado
- ½ c. of Brussels sprouts

DIRECTIONS

1. Split your Quinoa into 2 medium bowls.
2. Mix.
3. Top with your cucumber, avocado, and carrot.
4. Add the blanched Brussel Sprouts.
5. Serve and enjoy!

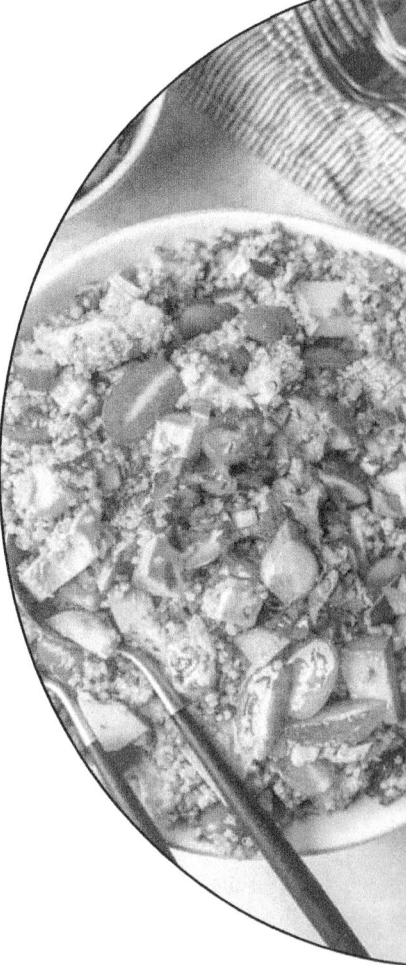

NUTRITION

- Calories: 472
- Protein: 11.2 g
- Carbs: 50.6 g
- Fat: 27.4 g

KALE SALAD WITH MIXED VEGETABLES

Preparation Time: 10 minutes
Cooking Time: 5 minutes
Servings: 2

INGREDIENTS

- 1 bunch of chopped Premier kale
- 1 c. of fresh peas
- 2 chopped carrots
- 1 c. of boiled potatoes
- 1 c. of sliced cabbage
- 2 tablespoons of apple cider vinegar
- 1 teaspoon of chili powder
- ½ teaspoon of salt
- 2 tablespoons of coconut oil
- 1 teaspoon of coconut powder

DIRECTIONS

1. Combine all vegetables with kale.
2. Drizzle with vinegar and coconut oil.
3. Season with salt and chili powder.
4. Sprinkle with coconut powder and toss to combine.
5. Add to a serving dish and serve. Enjoy.

NUTRITION

- Calories: 240
- Protein: 9 g
- Carbs: 36 g
- Fat: 9 g

CREAM OF CORN SOUP

Preparation Time: 5 minutes
Cooking Time: 15 minutes
Servings: 2

INGREDIENTS

- 0.5 lb. of corn puree
- 0.5 lb. of carrots
- 2 c. of vegetable stock
- ½ c. of chopped onion
- ½ teaspoon of salt
- ¼ teaspoon of pepper
- 1 teaspoon of dried thyme
- 2 oz. of chopped celery
- ½ tablespoon of olive oil
- 1 anise star

DIRECTIONS

1. Heat the olive oil in a medium pot and add onion; add celery, carrots and sauté for 15 minutes, until onion is caramelized.
2. Add the corn and stir until corn is tender.
3. Add the thyme and stir well.
4. Transfer the vegetables to a blender, add pumpkin puree, vegetable stock, and pulse until smooth.
5. Transfer the mixture into a sauce pan and simmer, add anise star and simmer over medium-high heat for 5-8 minutes or until heated through.
6. Remove the anise star and discard.
7. Serve immediately.

NUTRITION

- Calories: 223
- Protein: 7.84 g
- Carbs: 23.98 g
- Fat: 11.51 g

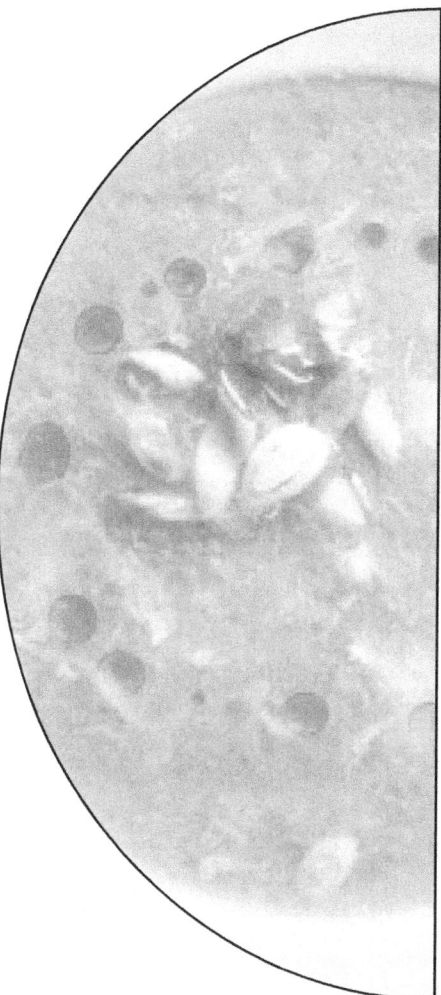

CLAM SOUP

Preparation Time: 15 minutes
Cooking Time: 5 minutes
Servings: 2

INGREDIENTS

- 1½ c. of water
- ½ fresh ginger
- 1 lb. of Manila clams
- 1 tablespoon of Chinese rice white wine
- ¼ teaspoon of salt
- ¼ teaspoon of white pepper

DIRECTIONS

1. In a large pot, boil water and add clams and ginger.
2. Cook until clams open, and then add wine.
3. Add the pepper and salt and serve hot.

NUTRITION

- Calories: 80
- Protein: 3 g
- Carbs: 16 g
- Fat: 0.5 g

APPLE & PEACH SALAD

Preparation Time: 3 minutes
Cooking Time: 5 minutes
Servings: 2

INGREDIENTS

- 2 chopped apples
- 1 c. of peach
- 1 c. of blackberries
- 1 tablespoon of lime juice
- 1 tablespoon of honey
- ¼ teaspoon of dried thyme
- ¼ teaspoon of sugar
- 1 teaspoon of salt

DIRECTIONS

1. Toss all ingredients together and put them into the serving dish.
2. Serve and enjoy.

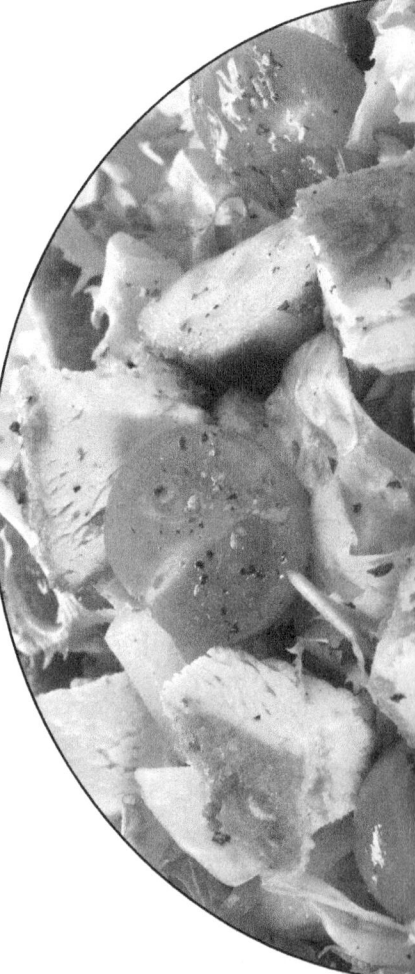

CHICKEN, APPLE & BASIL SALAD

Preparation Time: 6 minutes
Cooking Time: 5 minutes
Servings: 2

INGREDIENTS

- 4 c. of basil
- 2 c. of chopped apple
- 2 c. of chopped chicken breast
- ½ c. of sliced red onion
- ¼ c. of chopped pecans
- ¾ c. of Acai Dressing

DIRECTIONS

1. Set 4 salad bowls on the table and add basil to each.
2. Add each of your remaining ingredients as layers on top of the greens.
3. Once ready, drizzle each bowl of salad with 3 tablespoons of dressing.

CURRIED QUINOA SWEET POTATO SALAD

Preparation Time: 12 minutes
Cooking Time: 5 minutes
Servings: 2

INGREDIENTS

- 1 c. of curried quinoa
- 6 chopped sweet potatoes
- 1 c. of water
- ¼ c. of chopped onion
- 1 chopped celery
- Salt
- Pepper
- 3 boiled eggs
- 1 tablespoon of chopped dill
- ½ c. of mayonnaise
- 1 teaspoon of yellow mustard
- 1 teaspoon of vinegar

DIRECTIONS

1. Pour your potatoes and water into the cooker.
2. Securely close the lid and allow it to rise to high pressure over a high flame. Cook for about 3 minutes.
3. Remove the cooker from the flame and cool under cold running water.
4. Proceed to peel and dice potatoes, then layer them alternately with celery and onion.
5. Season with salt and pepper, then add your dill and chopped eggs.
6. In a separate bowl, combine the mustard, mayonnaise, and vinegar, folding the mixture gently into the potatoes.
7. Stir in your cooked quinoa.
8. Chill, serve, and enjoy!

NUTRITION

- Calories: 335.3
- Protein: 5.5 g
- Carbs: 55.2 g
- Fat: 9 g

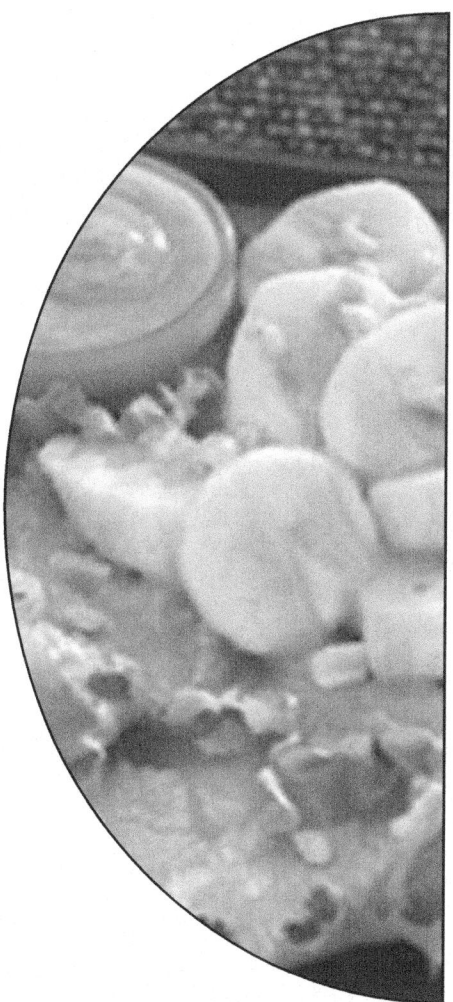

BANANA SALAD

Preparation Time: 5 minutes
Cooking Time: 5 minutes
Servings: 2

INGREDIENTS

- 4 sliced bananas
- ¼ c. of pineapple sauce
- 1 tablespoon of lime juice
- ¼ teaspoon of cinnamon powder
- ¼ teaspoon of chili flakes

DIRECTIONS

1. In a bowl, add bananas, pineapple sauce, lemon juice, and mix.
2. Now season with cinnamon and chili flakes.
3. Serve and enjoy.

NUTRITION

- Calories: 221
- Protein: 1.1 g
- Carbs: 57.5 g
- Fat: 0.3 g

CHAPTER 7.
DRESSINGS, SAUCES & SEASONING

PIZZA SAUCE

Preparation Time: 15 minutes
Cooking Time: 45 minutes
Servings: 2

INGREDIENTS

- 2 tablespoons of olive oil
- 2 anchovy fillets
- 2 tablespoons of fresh oregano leaves, finely chopped
- 3 garlic cloves, minced
- ½ teaspoon of dried oregano, crushed
- ½ teaspoon of red pepper flakes, crushed
- 1 -28-ounces can of whole peeled tomatoes, crushed
- ½ teaspoon of Erythritol
- Salt, as required
- Pinch of freshly ground black pepper
- Pinch of organic baking powder

DIRECTIONS

1. Heat the olive oil in a medium pan over medium-low heat and cook the anchovy fillets for about 1 minute, occasionally stirring.
2. Stir in the fresh oregano, garlic, dried oregano, and red pepper flakes and sauté for about 2-3 minutes.
3. Add the remaining ingredients except for baking powder and bring to a gentle simmer.
4. Reduce the heat to low and simmer for about 35-40 minutes, stirring occasionally.
5. Stir in the baking powder and remove it from heat.
6. Set aside at room temperature to cool completely before serving.
7. You can preserve this sauce in the refrigerator by placing it into an airtight container.

NUTRITION

- Calories: 56
- Net Carbs: 3.4 g
- Carbohydrates: 5.1 g
- Fiber: 1.7 g
- Protein: 1.4 g
- Fat: 4 g
- Sugar: 2.7 g
- Sodium: 61 mg

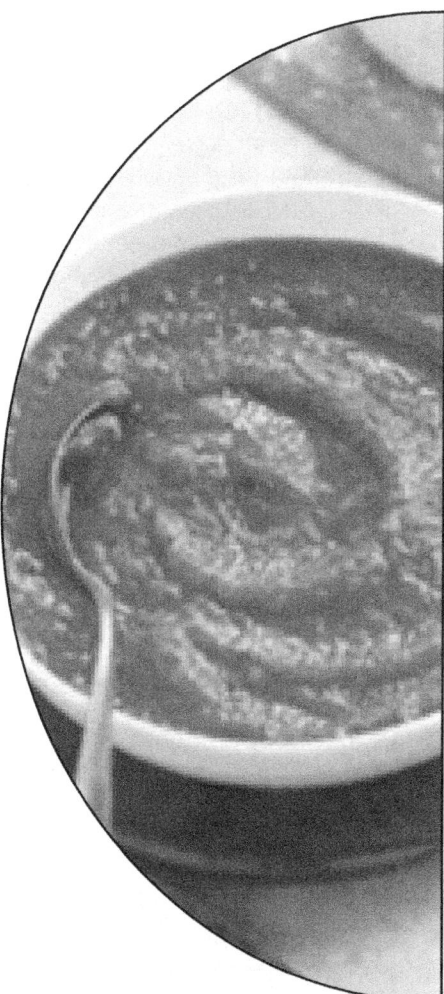

MARINARA SAUCE

Preparation Time: 10 minutes
Cooking Time: 5 minutes
Servings: 2

INGREDIENTS

- 2 tablespoons of olive oil
- 1 garlic clove
- 2 teaspoons of onion flakes
- 2 teaspoons of fresh thyme, finely chopped
- 2 teaspoons of fresh oregano, finely chopped
- 24 ounces of tomato puree
- 1 tablespoon of balsamic vinegar
- 2 teaspoons of Erythritol
- Salt and ground black pepper, as required
- 2 tablespoons of fresh parsley, finely chopped

DIRECTIONS

1. Heat the olive oil in a medium pan over medium-low heat and sauté the garlic, onion flakes, thyme, and oregano for about 3 minutes.
2. Stir in the tomato puree, vinegar, Erythritol, salt, and black pepper, and bring to a gentle simmer.
3. Remove the pan of sauce from heat and stir in the parsley.
4. Set aside at room temperature to cool completely before serving.
5. You can preserve this sauce in the refrigerator by placing it into an airtight container.

NUTRITION

- Calories: 36
- Net Carbs: 3.6 g
- Carbohydrates: 4.7 g
- Fiber: 1.1 g
- Protein: 0.9 g
- Fat: 2 g
- Sugar: 2.3 g
- Sodium: 168 mg

BBQ SAUCE

Preparation Time: 15 minutes
Cooking Time: 20 minutes
Servings: 2

INGREDIENTS

- 2½ -6-ounces cans of tomato paste
- ½ cup of organic apple cider vinegar
- 1/3 cup of powdered Erythritol
- 2 tablespoons of Worcestershire sauce
- 1 tablespoon of liquid hickory smoke
- 2 teaspoons of smoked paprika
- 1 teaspoon of garlic powder
- ½ teaspoon of onion powder
- Salt, as required
- ¼ teaspoon of red chili powder
- ¼ teaspoon of cayenne pepper
- 1½ cups of water

DIRECTIONS

1. Add all the ingredients except water in a pan and beat until well combined.
2. Add 1 cup of water and beat until combined.
3. Add the remaining water and beat until well combined.
4. Place the pan over medium-high heat and bring to a gentle boil.
5. Adjust the heat to medium-low and simmer, uncovered for about 20 minutes, stirring frequently.
6. Remove from the heat and set aside to cool slightly before serving.
7. You can preserve this sauce in the refrigerator by placing it into an airtight container.

NUTRITION

- Calories: 22
- Net Carbs: 3.7 g
- Carbohydrate: 4.7 g
- Fiber: 1 g
- Protein: 1 g
- Fat: 0.1 g
- Sugar: 3 g
- Sodium: 85 mg

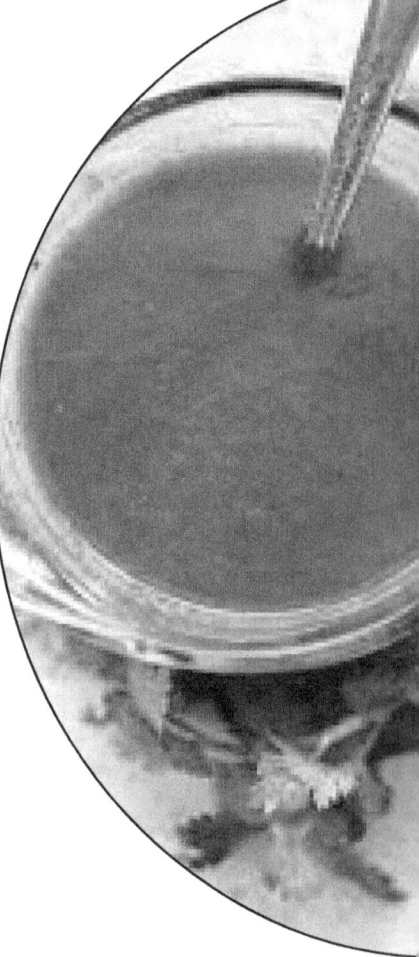

ENCHILADA SAUCE

Preparation Time: 10 minutes
Cooking Time: 10 minutes
Servings: 2

INGREDIENTS

- 3 ounces of salted butter
- 1½ tablespoons of Erythritol
- 2 teaspoons of dried oregano
- 3 teaspoons of ground cumin
- 2 teaspoons of ground coriander
- 2 teaspoons of onion powder
- ¼ teaspoon of cayenne pepper
- Salt and ground black pepper, as required
- 12 ounces of tomato puree

DIRECTIONS

1. Melt the butter in a medium pan over medium heat and sauté all the ingredients except tomato puree for about 3 minutes.
2. Add the tomato puree and simmer for about 5 minutes.
3. Remove the pan from heat and let it cool slightly before serving.
4. You can preserve this sauce in the refrigerator by placing it into an airtight container.
5. Note: you can add a little water if you prefer a thinner sauce.

NUTRITION

- Calories: 132
- Net Carbs: 5.1 g
- Carbohydrates: 6.6 g
- Fiber: 1.5 g
- Protein: 1.4 g
- Fat: 11.9 g
- Sugar: 3.1 g
- Sodium: 127 mg

TERIYAKI SAUCE

Preparation Time: 10 minutes
Cooking Time: 15 minutes
Servings: 2

INGREDIENTS

- ½ cup of low-sodium soy sauce
- 1 cup of water
- 2 tablespoons of organic apple cider vinegar
- ¼ cup of Erythritol
- 1 tablespoon of sesame oil
- ½ teaspoon of ginger powder
- 2 teaspoons of garlic powder
- ½ teaspoon of xanthan gum
- 2 teaspoons of sesame seeds

DIRECTIONS

1. Place all the ingredients except xanthan gum and sesame seeds in a small pan and mix well.
2. Now, place the pan over medium heat and bring it to a boil.
3. Sprinkle with the xanthan gum and beat until well combined.
4. Cook for about 8-10 minutes or until the sauce becomes thick.
5. Remove the pan from heat and mix in the sesame seeds.
6. Serve hot.
7. You can preserve this cooled sauce in the refrigerator by placing it into an airtight container.

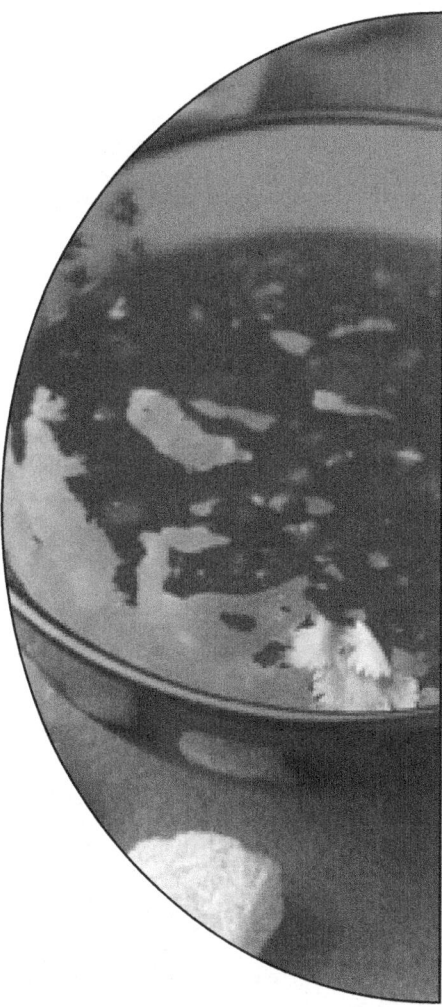

NUTRITION

- Calories: 29
- Net Carbs: 1.6 g
- Carbohydrates: 2 g
- Fiber: 0.4 g
- Protein: 1.3 g
- Fat: 2.1 g
- Sugar: 1.2 g
- Sodium: 886 mg

HOISIN SAUCE

Preparation Time: 10 minutes
Cooking Time: 0 minutes
Servings: 2

INGREDIENTS

- 4 tablespoons of low-sodium soy sauce
- 2 tablespoons of natural peanut butter
- 1 tablespoon of Erythritol
- 2 teaspoons of balsamic vinegar
- 2 teaspoons of sesame oil
- 1 teaspoon of Sriracha
- 1 garlic clove, peeled
- Ground black pepper, as required

DIRECTIONS

1. Add all the ingredients to a food processor and pulse until smooth.
2. You can preserve this sauce in the refrigerator by placing it into an airtight container.

NUTRITION

- Calories: 39
- Net Carbs: 1.2 g
- Carbohydrates: 1.5 g
- Fiber: 0.3 g
- Protein: 1.8 g
- Fat: 3.1 g
- Sugar: 0.8 g
- Sodium: 445 mg

HOT SAUCE

Preparation Time: 15 minutes
Cooking Time: 15 minutes
Servings: 2

INGREDIENTS

- 1 tablespoon of olive oil
- 1 cup of carrot, peeled and chopped
- ½ cup of yellow onion, chopped
- 5 garlic cloves, minced
- 6 habanero peppers, stemmed
- 1 tomato, chopped
- 1 tablespoon of fresh lemon zest
- ¼ cup of fresh lemon juice
- ¼ cup of balsamic vinegar
- ¼ cup of water
- Salt and ground black pepper, as required

DIRECTIONS

1. Heat the oil in a large pan over medium heat and cook the carrot, onion, and garlic for about 8-10 minutes, frequently stirring.
2. Remove the pan from heat and let it cool slightly.
3. Place the onion mixture and the remaining ingredients in a food processor and pulse until smooth.
4. Return the mixture into the same pan over medium-low heat and simmer for about 3-5 minutes, stirring occasionally.
5. Remove the pan from heat and let it cool completely.
6. You can preserve this sauce in the refrigerator by placing it into an airtight container.

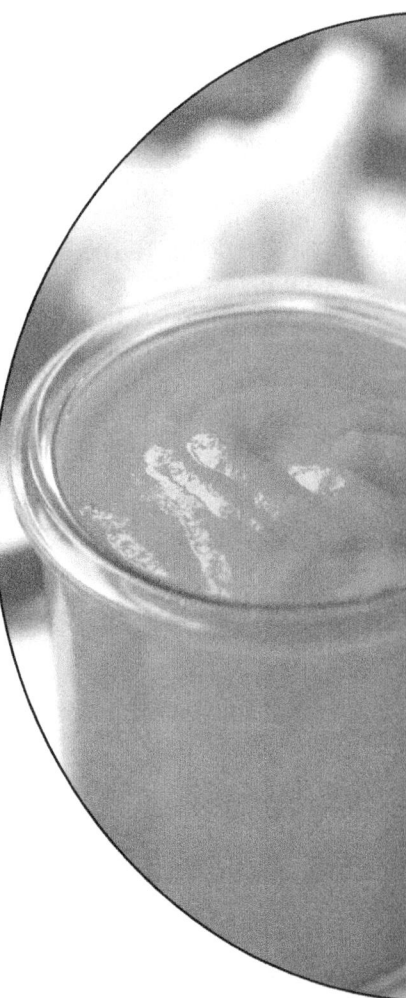

NUTRITION

- Calories: 9
- Net Carbs: 1 g
- Carbohydrates: 1.3 g
- Fiber: 0.3 g
- Protein: 0.2 g
- Fat: 0.4 g
- Sugar: 0.7 g
- Sodium: 7 mg

WORCESTERSHIRE SAUCE

Preparation Time: 5 minutes
Cooking Time: 5 minutes
Servings: 2

INGREDIENTS

- ½ cup of organic apple cider vinegar
- 2 tablespoons of low-sodium soy sauce
- 2 tablespoons of water
- ¼ teaspoon of ground mustard
- ¼ teaspoon of ground ginger
- ¼ teaspoon of garlic powder
- ¼ teaspoon of onion powder
- 1/8 teaspoon of ground cinnamon
- 1/8 teaspoon of ground black pepper

DIRECTIONS

1. Add all the ingredients to a small pan and mix well.
2. Now, place the pan over medium heat and bring it to a boil.
3. Adjust the heat to low and simmer for about 1-2 minutes.
4. Remove the pan from heat and let it cool completely.
5. You can preserve this sauce in the refrigerator by placing it into an airtight container.

NUTRITION

- Calories: 5
- Net Carbs: 0.4 g
- Carbohydrates: 0.5 g
- Fiber: 0.1 g
- Protein: 0.2 g
- Fat: 0 g
- Sugar: 0.3 g
- Sodium: 177 mg

ALMOND BUTTER

Preparation Time: 15 minutes
Cooking Time: 15 minutes
Servings: 2

INGREDIENTS

- 2¼ cups of raw almonds
- 1 tablespoon of coconut oil
- ¾ teaspoon of salt
- 4-6 drops of liquid stevia
- ½ teaspoon of ground cinnamon

DIRECTIONS

1. Preheat the oven to 325 ºF.
2. Arrange the almonds onto a rimmed baking sheet in an even layer.
3. Bake for about 12-15 minutes.
4. Remove the almonds from the oven and let them cool completely.
5. In a food processor fitted with a metal blade, place the almonds and pulse until a fine meal forms.
6. Add the coconut oil, salt, and pulse for about 6-9 minutes.
7. Add the stevia, cinnamon, and pulse for about 1-2 minutes.
8. You can preserve this almond butter in the refrigerator by placing it into an airtight container.

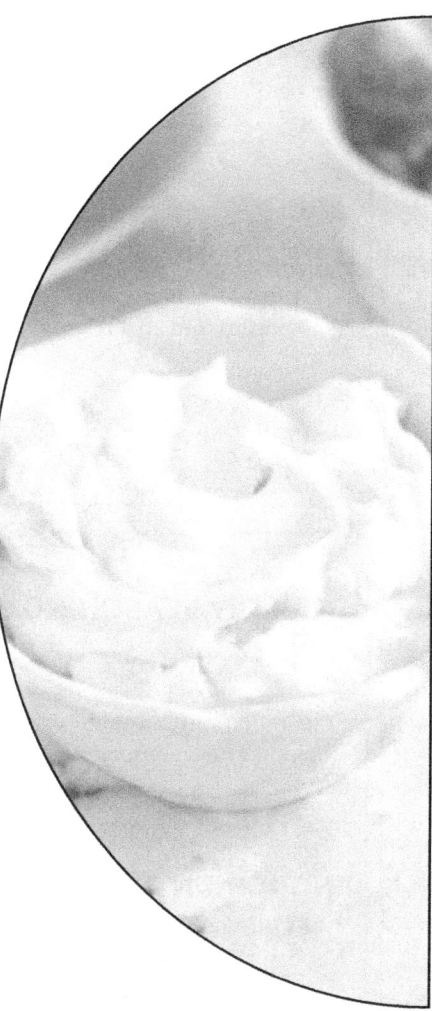

MAYONNAISE

Preparation Time: 10 minutes
Cooking Time: 0 minutes
Servings: 2

INGREDIENTS

- 2 organic egg yolks
- 3 teaspoons of fresh lemon juice, divided
- 1 teaspoon of mustard
- ½ cup of coconut oil, melted
- ½ cup of olive oil
- Salt and ground black pepper, as required -optional

DIRECTIONS

1. Place the egg yolks, 1 teaspoon of lemon juice, and mustard in a blender and pulse until combined.
2. While the motor is running gradually, add both oils and pulse until a thick mixture forms.
3. Add the remaining lemon juice, salt, and black pepper and pulse until well combined.
4. You can preserve this mayonnaise in the refrigerator by placing into an airtight container.
5. Note: if the mayonnaise seems too thin, slowly add more oils while the motor is running until thick.

SEASONED SALT

Preparation Time: 5 minutes
Cooking Time: 0 minutes
Servings: 28

INGREDIENTS

- ¼ cup of kosher salt
- ½ teaspoon of onion powder
- 1 teaspoon of garlic powder
- 1 teaspoon of paprika
- ½ teaspoon of ground red pepper
- 4 teaspoons of freshly ground black pepper

DIRECTIONS

1. Add all the ingredients to a bowl and stir to combine.
2. Transfer into an airtight jar to preserve.

NUTRITION

- Calories: 2
- Net Carbs: 0.4 g
- Carbohydrates: 0.6 g
- Fiber: 0.2 g
- Protein: 0.1 g
- Fat: 0.1 g
- Sugar: 0.1 g
- Sodium: 1500 mg

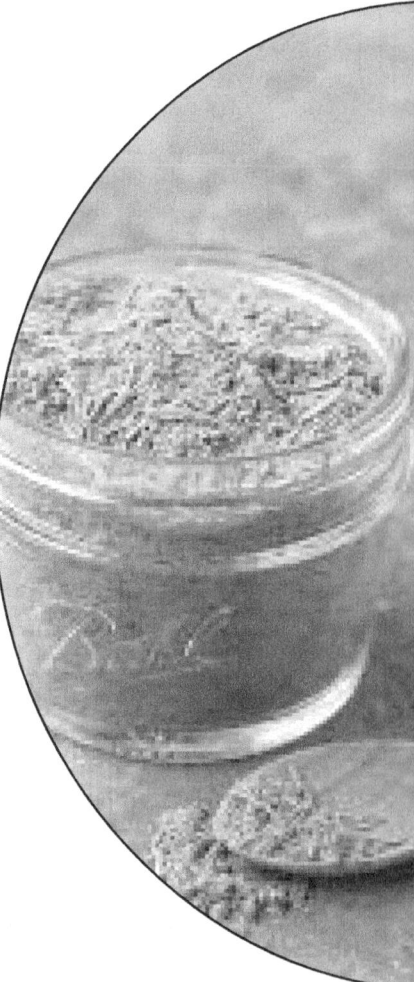

POULTRY SEASONING

Preparation Time: 5 minutes
Cooking Time: 0 minutes
Servings: 2

INGREDIENTS

- 2 teaspoons of dried sage, crushed finely
- 1 teaspoon of dried marjoram, crushed finely
- ¾ teaspoon of dried rosemary, crushed finely
- 1½ teaspoons of dried thyme, crushed finely
- ½ teaspoon of ground nutmeg
- ½ teaspoon of ground black pepper

DIRECTIONS

1. 1. Add all the ingredients to a bowl and stir to combine.
2. 2. Transfer into an airtight jar to preserve.

NUTRITION

- Calories: 2
- Net Carbs: 0.2 g
- Carbohydrates: 0.4 g
- Fiber: 0.2 g
- Protein: 0.1 g
- Fat: 0.1 g
- Sugar: 0 g
- Sodium: 0 mg

TACO SEASONING

Preparation Time: 5 minutes
Cooking Time: 0 minutes
Servings: 2

INGREDIENTS

- ½ teaspoon of dried oregano, crushed
- ½ teaspoon of ground cumin
- 2 teaspoons of hot chili powder
- 1½ teaspoons of paprika
- Pinch of red pepper flakes, crushed
- Pinch of cayenne pepper
- ¼ teaspoon of ground black pepper
- 1 teaspoon of onion powder
- ½ teaspoon of garlic powder
- ½ teaspoon of sea salt

DIRECTIONS

1. Add all the ingredients to a bowl and stir to combine.
2. Transfer into an airtight jar to preserve.

NUTRITION

- Net Carbs: 0.5 g
- Carbohydrates: 0.8 g
- Fiber: 0.3 g
- Protein: 0.2 g
- Fat: 0.1 g
- Sugar: 0.2 g
- Sodium: 83 mg

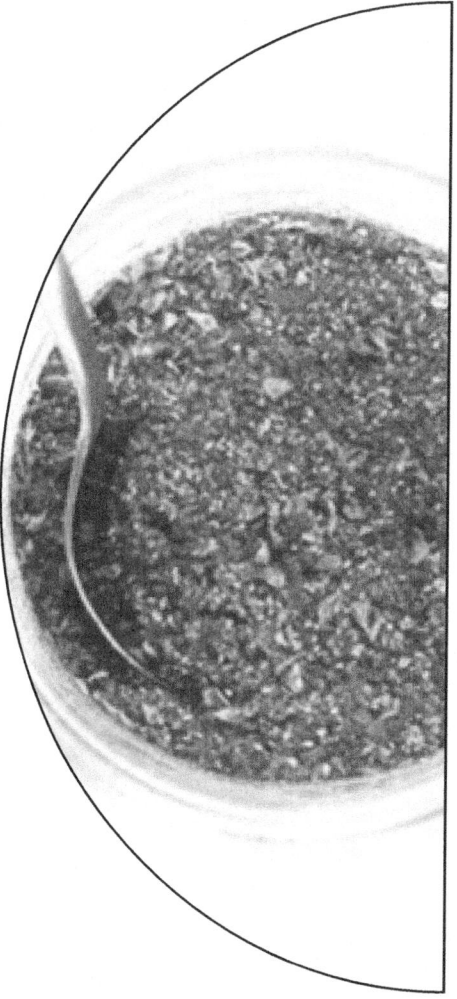

PUMPKIN PIE SPICE

Preparation Time: 5 minutes
Cooking Time: 0 minutes
Servings: 2

INGREDIENTS

- 1 teaspoon of ground cinnamon
- ¼ teaspoon of ground ginger
- ¼ teaspoon of ground nutmeg
- 1/8 teaspoon of ground cloves

DIRECTIONS

1. Add all the ingredients to a bowl and stir to combine.
2. Transfer into an airtight jar to preserve.

NUTRITION

- Calories: 4
- Net Carbs: 0.4 g
- Carbohydrates: 0.9 g
- Fiber: 0.5 g
- Protein: 0.1 g
- Fat: 0.1 g
- Sugar: 0.1 g
- Sodium: 0 mg

CURRY POWDER

Preparation Time: 10 minutes
Cooking Time: 10 minutes
Servings: 2

INGREDIENTS

- ¼ cup of coriander seeds
- 2 tablespoons of mustard seeds
- 2 tablespoons of cumin seeds
- 2 tablespoons of anise seeds
- 1 tablespoon of whole allspice berries
- 1 tablespoon of fenugreek seeds
- 5 tablespoons of ground turmeric

DIRECTIONS

1. In a large nonstick frying pan, place all the spices except turmeric over medium heat and cook for about 9-10 minutes or until toasted completely, stirring continuously.
2. Remove the frying pan from heat and set it aside to cool.
3. In a spice grinder, add the toasted spices and turmeric and grind until a fine powder forms.
4. Transfer into an airtight jar to preserve.

NUTRITION

- Calories: 19
- Net Carbs: 0.6 g
- Carbohydrates: 2.4 g
- Fiber: 1.8 g
- Protein: 0.8 g
- Fat: 0.8 g
- Sugar: 0.1 g
- Sodium: 2 mg

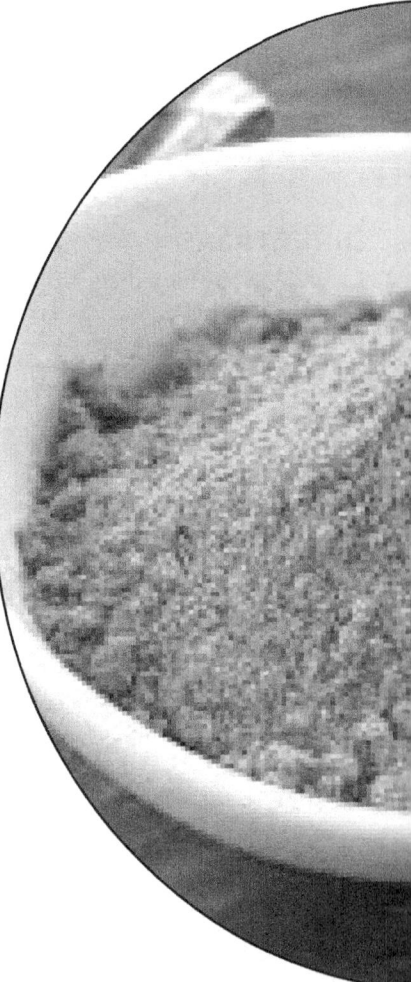

CHAPTER 8.

SNACKS

ONION AND CAULIFLOWER DIP

Preparation Time: 10 minutes
Cooking Time: 40 minutes
Servings: 2

NUTRITION

- Calories: 60
- Fat: 4 g
- Fiber: 1 g
- Carbs: 1 g
- Protein: 1 g

INGREDIENTS

- 1 cauliflower head, florets separated
- 1½ cups of chicken stock
- 1/2 teaspoon of chili powder
- 1/2 teaspoon of garlic powder
- 1/4 cup of mayonnaise
- 1/2 cup of yellow onion, chopped.
- 1/2 teaspoon of cumin, ground
- ¾ cup of cream cheese
- Salt and black pepper to the taste

DIRECTIONS

1. Put the stock in a pot, add cauliflower and onion, heat up over medium heat and cook for 30 minutes.
2. Add the chili powder, salt, pepper, cumin, and garlic powder and stir.
3. Also, add the cream cheese and stir a bit until it melts
4. Blend using an immersion blender and mix with the mayo.
5. Transfer to a bowl and keep in the fridge for 2 hours before you serve it.

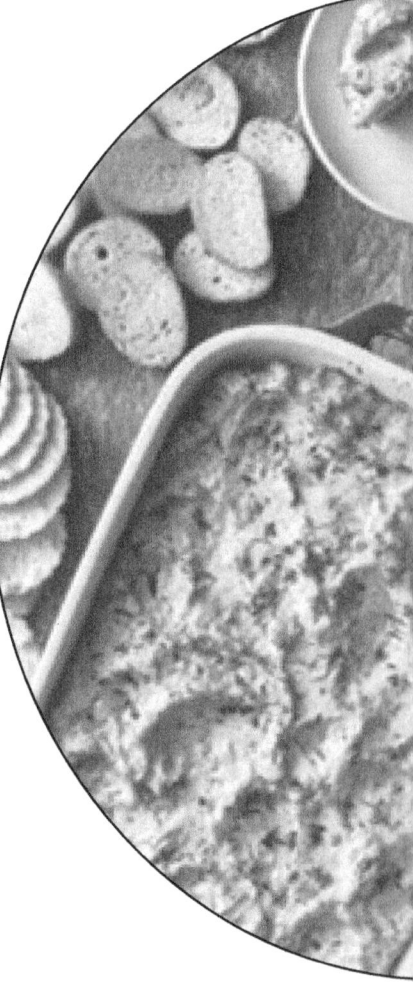

DELIGHTFUL BOMBS

Preparation Time: 10 minutes
Cooking Time: 10 minutes
Servings: 2

INGREDIENTS
- 8 black olives, pitted and chopped
- 4 ounces of cream cheese
- 1 tablespoon of basil, chopped
- 2 tablespoons of sun-dried tomato pesto
- 14 pepperoni slices, chopped
- Salt and black pepper to the taste

DIRECTIONS
1. In a bowl, mix cream cheese with salt, pepper, pepperoni, basil, sun-dried tomato pesto, and black olives and stir well.
2. Shape balls from this mix, arrange on a platter and serve.

NUTRITION

- Calories: 110
- Fat: 10 g
- Fiber: 0 g
- Carbs: 1.4 g
- Protein: 3 g

PESTO CRACKERS

Preparation Time: 27 minutes
Cooking Time: 20 minutes
Servings: 2

INGREDIENTS

- 1/2 teaspoon of baking powder
- 1/4 teaspoon of basil, dried
- 1¼ cups of almond flour
- 1 garlic clove, minced
- 2 tablespoons of basil pesto
- A pinch of cayenne pepper
- 3 tablespoons of ghee
- Salt and black pepper to the taste.

DIRECTIONS

1. In a bowl, mix salt, pepper, baking powder, and almond flour.
2. Add the garlic, cayenne, and basil and stir.
3. Add the pesto and whisk.
4. Also, add the ghee and mix your dough with your finger.
5. Spread this dough on a lined baking sheet, introduce in the oven at 325 °F and bake for 17 minutes.
6. Leave it aside to cool down, cut your crackers and serve them as a snack.

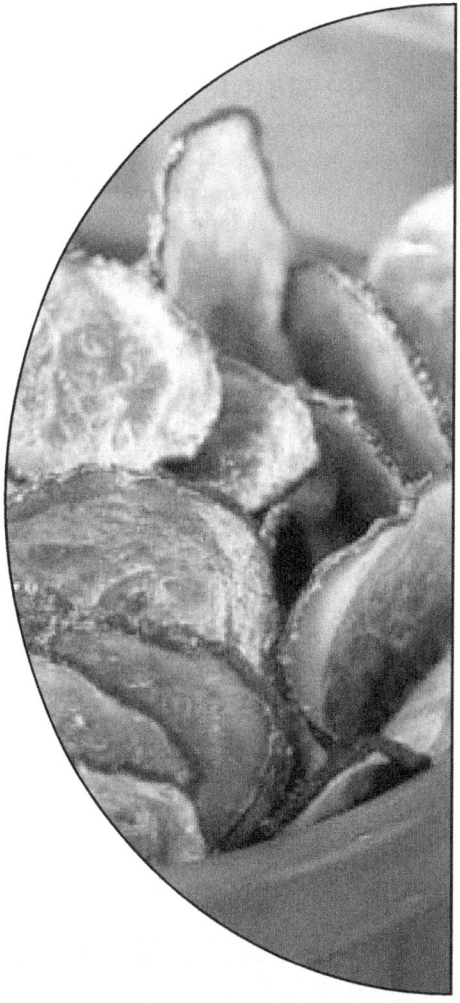

ZUCCHINI CHIPS

Preparation Time: 10 minutes
Cooking Time: 3 hours 10 minutes
Servings: 2

INGREDIENTS

- 3 zucchinis, very thinly sliced
- 2 tablespoons of balsamic vinegar
- 2 tablespoons of olive oil
- Salt and black pepper to the taste

DIRECTIONS

1. In a bowl, mix oil with vinegar, salt, and pepper and whisk well.
2. Add the zucchini slices, toss to coat well and spread on a lined baking sheet, introduce in the oven at 200 °F and bake for 3 hours
3. Leave chips to cool down and serve them as a snack.

AVOCADO DIP

Preparation Time: 3 hours 20 minutes
Cooking Time: 10 minutes
Servings: 2

INGREDIENTS

- 2 avocados, pitted, peeled, and cut into slices
- 1/2 cup of cilantro, chopped.
- 1 cup of coconut milk
- 1/4 cup of Erythritol powder
- 1/4 teaspoon of stevia
- Juice and zest of 2 limes

DIRECTIONS

1. Place the avocado slices on a lined baking sheet, squeeze half of the lime juice over them and keep in your freezer for 3 hours.
2. Heat the coconut milk in a pan over medium heat.
3. Add the lime zest; stir, and bring to a boil.
4. Add the Erythritol powder; stir, take off the heat and leave aside to cool down a bit.
5. Transfer avocado to your food processor, add the rest of the lime juice and the cilantro and pulse well.
6. Add the coconut milk mix and stevia and blend well.
7. Transfer to a bowl and serve right away.

NUTRITION

- Calories: 150
- Fat: 14 g
- Fiber: 2 g
- Carbs: 4 g
- Protein: 2 g

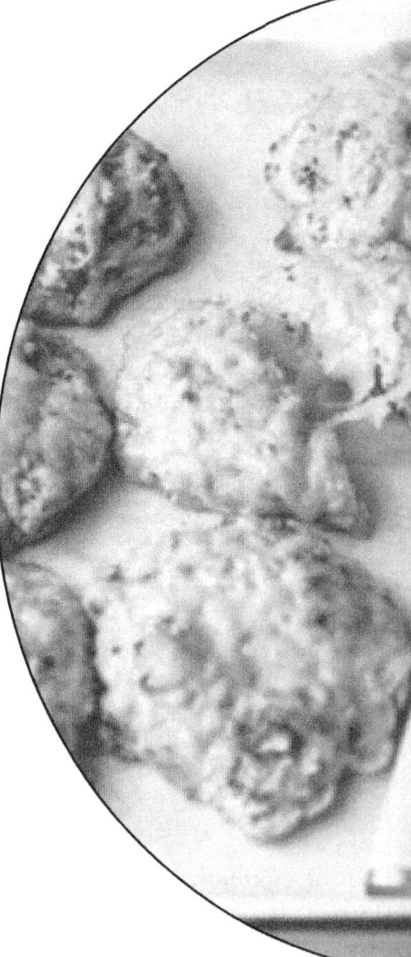

BROCCOLI AND CHEDDAR BISCUITS

Preparation Time: 35 minutes
Cooking Time: 20 minutes
Servings: 2

INGREDIENTS

- 4 cups of broccoli florets
- 1½ cup of almond flour
- 2 eggs
- 1/2 teaspoon of apple cider vinegar
- 1/2 teaspoon of baking soda
- 1 teaspoon of paprika
- 1/4 cup of coconut oil
- 2 cups of cheddar cheese, grated
- 1 teaspoon of garlic powder
- Salt and black pepper to the taste.

DIRECTIONS

1. Put the broccoli florets in your food processor, add some salt and pepper and blend well.
2. In a bowl, mix almond flour with salt, pepper, paprika, garlic powder, and baking soda and stir.
3. Add the cheddar cheese, coconut oil, eggs, vinegar, and stir everything.
4. Add the broccoli and stir again.
5. Shape 12 patties, arrange on a baking sheet, introduce in the oven at 375 ºF and bake for 20 minutes.
6. Turn the oven to broiler and broil your biscuits for 5 minutes more
7. Arrange on a platter and serve

NUTRITION

- Calories: 163
- Fat: 12 g
- Fiber: 2 g
- Carbs: 2 g
- Protein: 7 g

CELERY STICKS

Preparation Time: 10 minutes
Cooking Time: 10 minutes
Servings: 2

INGREDIENTS

- 2 cups of rotisserie chicken, shredded
- 6 celery sticks cut in halves
- 3 tablespoons of hot tomato sauce
- 1/4 cup of mayonnaise
- 1/2 teaspoon of garlic powder
- Some chopped chives for serving
- Salt and black pepper to the taste

DIRECTIONS

1. In a bowl, mix chicken with salt, pepper, garlic powder, mayo, tomato sauce and stir well.
2. Arrange the celery pieces on a platter, spread chicken mix over them, sprinkle some chives, and serve.

NUTRITION

- Calories: 100
- Fat: 2 g
- Fiber: 3 g
- Carbs: 1 g
- Protein: 6 g

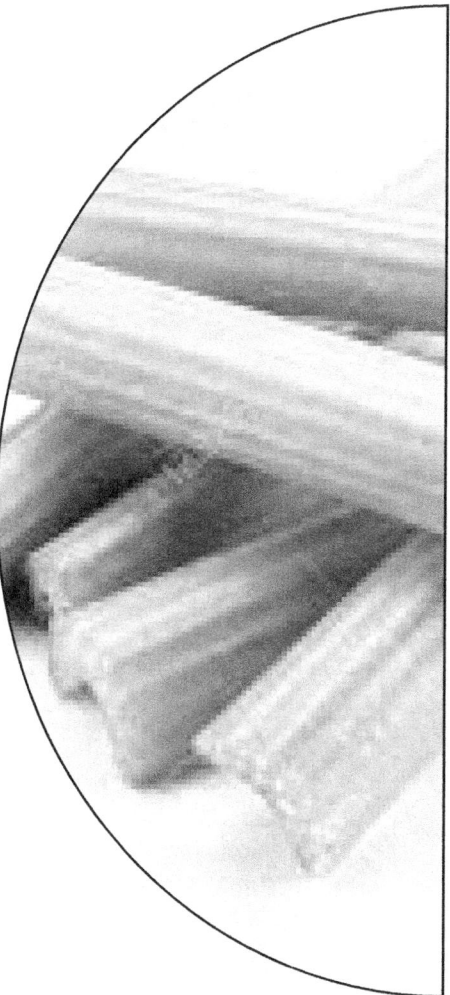

DELIGHTFUL CUCUMBER CUPS

Preparation Time: 10 minutes
Cooking Time: 10 minutes
Servings: 2

INGREDIENTS

- 2 cucumbers, peeled, cut into ¾ inch slices, and some of the seeds scooped out
- 1/2 cup of sour cream
- 2 teaspoons of lime juice
- 1 tablespoon of lime zest
- 6 ounces of smoked salmon, flaked
- 1/3 cup of cilantro, chopped.
- A pinch of cayenne pepper
- Salt and white pepper to the taste

DIRECTIONS

1. In a bowl, mix salmon with salt, pepper, cayenne, sour cream, lime juice and zest, cilantro and stir well.
2. Fill each cucumber cup with this salmon mix, arrange on a platter and serve as an appetizer.

NUTRITION

- Calories: 30
- Fat: 11 g
- Fiber: 1 g
- Carbs: 1 g
- Protein: 2 g

EGG CHIPS

Preparation Time: 15 minutes
Cooking Time: 15 minutes
Servings: 2

INGREDIENTS

- 4 eggs whites
- 2 tablespoons of parmesan, shredded
- 1/2 tablespoon of water
- Salt and black pepper to the taste

DIRECTIONS

1. In a bowl, mix the egg whites with salt, pepper, and water and whisk well.
2. Spoon this into a muffin pan, sprinkle cheese on top, introduce in the oven at 400 °F and bake for 15 minutes.
3. Transfer the egg white chips to a platter and serve with a dip on the side.

NUTRITION

- Calories: 120
- Fat: 2 g
- Fiber: 1 g
- Carbs: 2 g
- Protein: 7 g

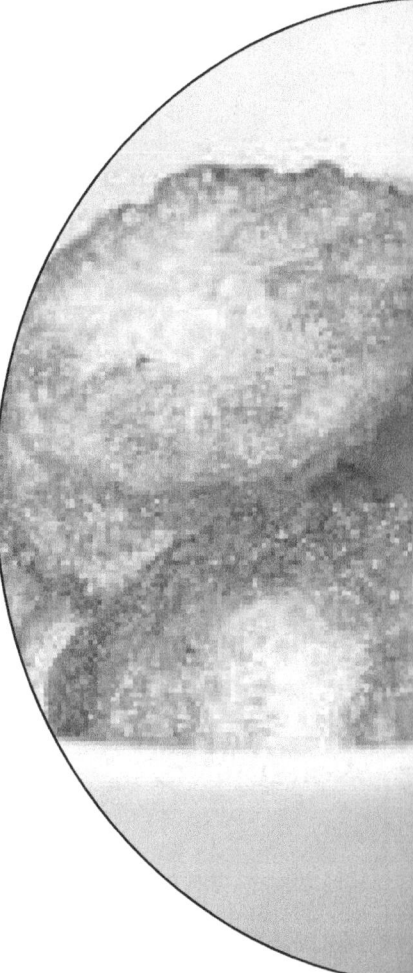

CHEESE BURGER MUFFINS

Preparation Time: 40 minutes
Cooking Time: 20 minutes
Servings: 2

INGREDIENTS

- 1/2 cup of flaxseed meal
- 1 teaspoon of baking powder
- 1/4 cups of sour cream
- 1/2 cup of almond flour
- 2 eggs
- Salt and black pepper to the taste

For the filling:
- 1/2 teaspoon of onion powder
- 2 tablespoons of tomato paste
- 1/2 teaspoon of garlic powder
- 1/2 cup of cheddar cheese, grated
- 16 ounces of beef, ground
- 2 tablespoons of mustard
- Salt and black pepper to the taste

DIRECTIONS

1. In a bowl, mix almond flour with a flaxseed meal, salt, pepper, baking powder, and whisk.
2. Add the eggs and sour cream and stir very well.
3. Divide this into a greased muffin pan and press well using your fingers.
4. Heat a pan over medium-high heat; add beef; stir and brown for a few minutes.
5. Add salt, pepper, onion powder, garlic powder, and tomato paste and stir well.
6. Cook for 5 minutes more and take off the heat.
7. Fill the cupcakes crusts with this mix, introduce in the oven at 350 °F and bake for 15 minutes.
8. Spread cheese on top, introduce in the oven again and bake muffins for 5 minutes more.
9. Serve with mustard and your favorite toppings on top.

NUTRITION

- Calories: 245
- Fat: 16 g
- Fiber: 6 g
- Carbs: 2 g
- Protein: 14 g

TOMATO TARTS

Preparation Time: 10 minutes
Cooking Time: 1 hour 20 minutes
Servings: 2

INGREDIENTS

- 2 tomatoes, sliced
- 1/4 cup of olive oil
- Salt and black pepper to the taste

For the base:
- 5 tablespoons of ghee
- 1 tablespoon of psyllium husk
- 1/2 cup of almond flour
- 2 tablespoons of coconut flour
- A pinch of salt

For the filling:
- 3 ounces of goat cheese, crumbled
- 1 small onion, thinly sliced
- 3 teaspoons of thyme, chopped
- 2 tablespoons of olive oil
- 2 teaspoons of garlic, minced

DIRECTIONS

1. Spread the tomato slices on a lined baking sheet, season with salt and pepper, drizzle 1/4 cup of olive oil, introduce in the oven at 425 °F and bake for 40 minutes.
2. Meanwhile, in your food processor, mix the almond flour with psyllium husk, coconut flour, salt, pepper, ghee, and stir until you obtain a dough.
3. Divide this dough into silicone cupcake molds, press well, introduce in the oven at 350 °F and bake for 20 minutes.
4. Take cupcakes out of the oven and leave them aside.
5. Also, take tomato slices out of the oven and cool them down a bit.
6. Divide the tomato slices on top of cupcakes.
7. Heat a pan with 2 tablespoons of olive oil over medium-high heat; add onion; stir, and cook for 4 minutes.
8. Add the garlic and thyme; stir, cook for 1 minute more and take off the heat.
9. Spread this mix on top of tomato slices.
10. Sprinkle goat cheese, introduce in the oven again and cook at 350 °F for 5 more minutes.
11. Arrange on a platter and serve.

NUTRITION
- Calories: 163
- Fat: 13 g
- Fiber: 1 g
- Carbs: 3 g
- Protein: 3 g

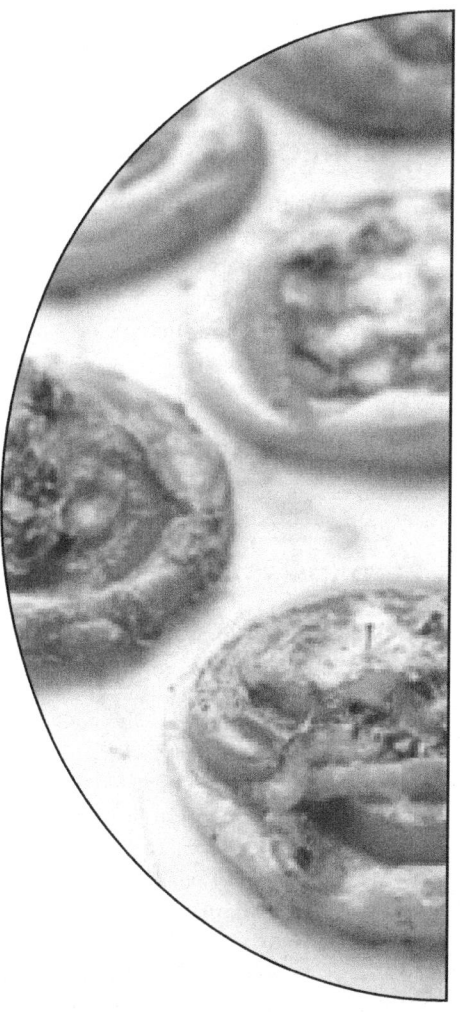

PIZZA DIP

Preparation Time: 30 minutes
Cooking Time: 20 minutes
Servings: 2

INGREDIENTS

- 4 ounces of cream cheese, soft
- 1/2 cup of tomato sauce
- 1/4 cup of mayonnaise
- 1/2 cup of mozzarella cheese
- 6 pepperoni slices, chopped
- 1/2 teaspoon of Italian seasoning
- 1/4 cup of sour cream
- 1/4 cup of parmesan cheese, grated
- 1 tablespoon of green bell pepper, chopped
- 4 black olives, pitted and chopped
- Salt and black pepper, to the taste

DIRECTIONS

1. In a bowl, mix the cream cheese with mozzarella, sour cream, mayo, salt, pepper and stir well.
2. Spread this into 4 ramekins. Add a layer of tomato sauce, then a layer parmesan cheese. Top with bell pepper, pepperoni, Italian seasoning, and black olives.
3. Introduce in the oven at 350 °F and bake for 20 minutes.
4. Serve warm.

NUTRITION
- Calories: 400
- Fat: 34 g
- Fiber: 4 g
- Carbs: 4 g
- Protein: 15 g

PROSCIUTTO AND SHRIMP APPETIZER

Preparation Time: 30 minutes
Cooking Time: 15 minutes
Servings: 2

INGREDIENTS

- 11 prosciutto sliced
- 10 ounces of already cooked shrimp, peeled and deveined
- 2 tablespoons of olive oil
- 1/3 cup of blackberries, ground
- 1/3 cup of red wine
- 1 tablespoon of mint, chopped.
- 2 tablespoons of Erythritol

DIRECTIONS

1. Wrap each shrimp in prosciutto slices, arrange on a lined baking sheet, drizzle the olive oil over them, introduce in the oven at 425 °F and bake for 15 minutes.
2. Heat a pan with ground blackberries over medium heat; add mint, wine, Erythritol; stir, cook for 3 minutes and take off the heat.
3. Arrange the shrimps on a platter; drizzle blackberries sauce over them and serve.

NUTRITION

- Calories: 245
- Fat: 12 g
- Fiber: 2 g
- Carbs: 1 g
- Protein: 14 g

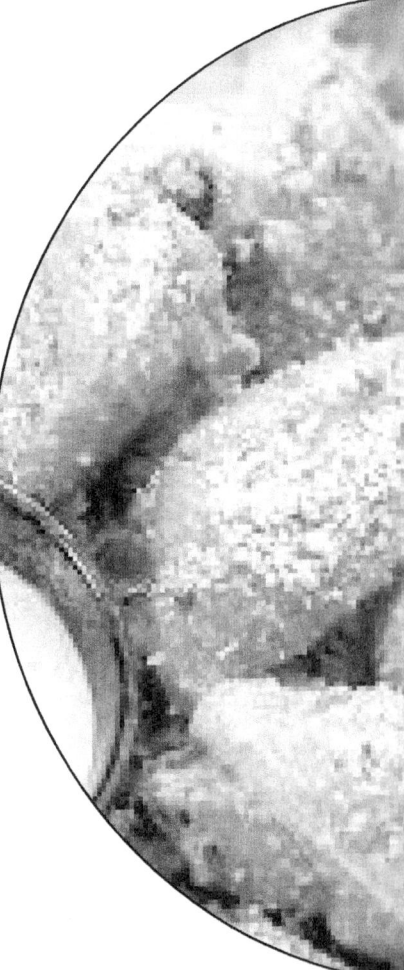

PARMESAN WINGS

Preparation Time: 34 minutes
Cooking Time: 25 minutes
Servings: 2

INGREDIENTS

- 6-pound of chicken wings, cut in halves
- 1/2 teaspoon of Italian seasoning
- 2 tablespoons of ghee
- 1/2 cup of parmesan cheese, grated
- 1 teaspoon of garlic powder
- 1 egg
- A pinch of red pepper flakes, crushed
- Salt and black pepper to the taste

DIRECTIONS

1. Arrange the chicken wings on a lined baking sheet. Introduce them in the oven at 425 ° F and bake for 17 minutes.
2. Meanwhile, in your blender, mix the ghee with cheese, egg, salt, pepper, pepper flakes, garlic powder, and Italian seasoning and blend very well.
3. Take the chicken wings out of the oven, flip them, turn the oven to broil, and broil them for 5 minutes more.
4. Take the chicken pieces out of the oven again, pour sauce over them, toss to coat well, and broil for 1 minute more.
5. Serve them as a quick appetizer.

NUTRITION

- Calories: 134
- Fat: 8 g
- Fiber: 1 g
- Carbs: 0.5 g
- Protein: 14 g

CHAPTER 9.
DESSERTS

COCONUT SPICED APPLE SMOOTHIE

Preparation Time: 5 minutes
Cooking Time: 10 minutes
Servings: 2

INGREDIENTS

- 1 apple
- 2 tablespoons of almond butter
- ¼ teaspoon of cinnamon powder
- 1 pinch of ground ginger
- 2 tablespoons of hemp seeds
- 2 tablespoons of honey
- 1 cup of coconut milk

DIRECTIONS

1. Start by preparing all the ingredients together, combining them in your blender, then pulse until smooth and well blended.
2. Pour the smoothies in tall glasses.
3. Serve and enjoy!

NUTRITION

- Calories: 123
- Fat: 14.6 g
- Fiber: 0.8 g
- Carbs: 8.6 g
- Protein: 4.6 g

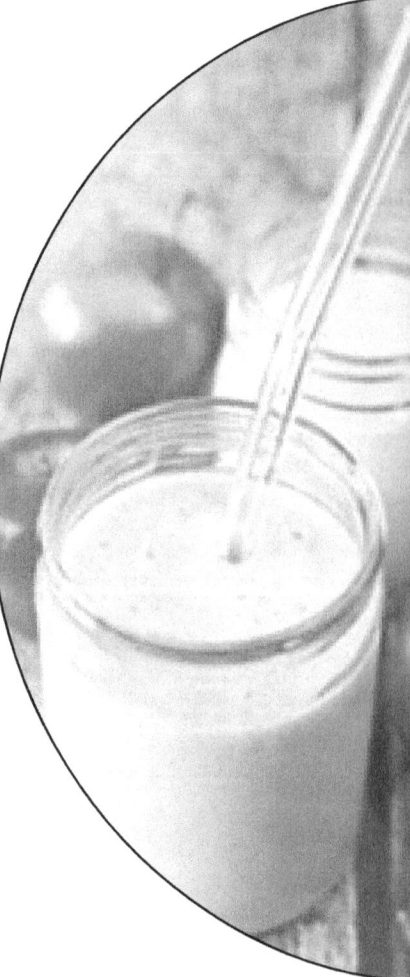

SWEET AND NUTTY SMOOTHIE

Preparation Time: 5 minutes
Cooking Time: 10 minutes
Servings: 2

INGREDIENTS

- 1 banana
- ½ cucumbers
- 1 tablespoon of peanut butter

DIRECTIONS

1. Start by preparing all the ingredients together, combining them in your blender, then pulse until smooth and well blended.
2. Pour the smoothies in tall glasses.
3. Serve and enjoy!

NUTRITION

- Calories: 121
- Fat: 14.6 g
- Fiber: 0.8 g
- Carbs: 8.6 g
- Protein: 4.6 g

ORANGE AND PEACHES SMOOTHIE

Preparation Time: 5 minutes
Cooking Time: 10 minutes
Servings: 2

INGREDIENTS

- 2 oranges, cut into segments
- 2 peaches, pitted and sliced
- 1 cup of carrot juice
- ¼ teaspoon of cinnamon powder
- 1 pinch of ground ginger
- 2 tablespoons of ground flaxseeds
- 1 tablespoon of chia seeds

DIRECTIONS

1. Start by preparing all the ingredients together, combining them in your blender, then pulse until smooth and well blended.
2. Pour the smoothies in tall glasses.
3. Serve and enjoy!

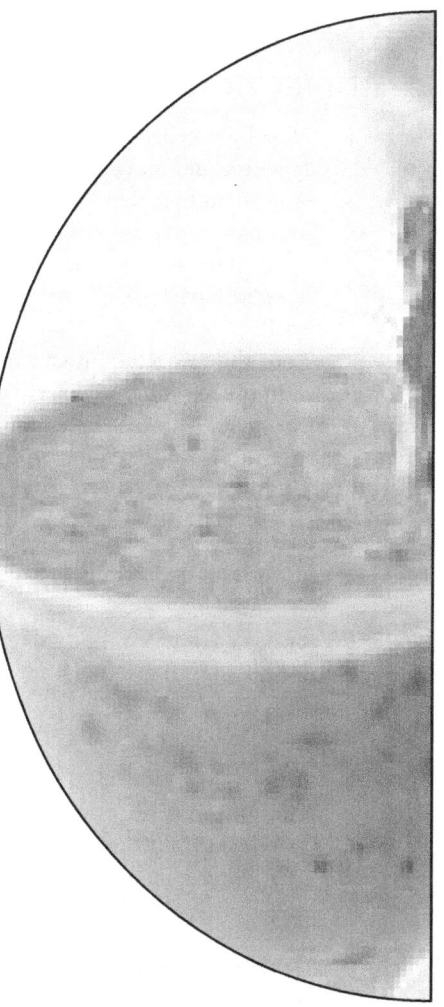

GINGER BERRY SMOOTHIE

Preparation Time: 5 minutes
Cooking Time: 10 minutes
Servings: 2

INGREDIENTS

- ½ cup of unsweetened almond milk
- 1 cup of mixed berries
- ½ cup of unsweetened plain yogurt
- 1 piece of fresh ginger, minced
- 4 or 5 ice cubes

DIRECTIONS

1. Start by preparing all the ingredients together, combining them in your blender, then pulse until smooth and well blended.
2. Pour the smoothies in tall glasses.
3. Serve and enjoy!

VEGETARIAN-FRIENDLY SMOOTHIE

Preparation Time: 5 minutes
Cooking Time: 10 minutes
Servings: 2

INGREDIENTS

- 950 ml of water
- 180 g of romaine lettuce
- 60 g of pineapple, chopped
- 2 tablespoons of fresh parsley
- 1 tablespoon of minced ginger
- 180 g of cucumber, peeled and finely chopped
- ½ cup of kiwi fruit, peeled and sliced
- ½ avocado, sliced
- 1 tablespoon of sugar substitute
- Ice cubes for serving

DIRECTIONS

1. Start by preparing all the ingredients together, then wash the lettuce leaves properly with water and coarsely chop it using a knife.
2. Add them to a blender. To this, add chopped pineapple, ginger, cucumber, kiwi, avocado, sugar substitute, and water.
3. Give all the ingredients a whisk. Now add some parsley and blend the mixture into a smooth paste. Make sure there are no lumps. You can also strain this juice if you wish.
4. Pour the smoothie into a large glass.
5. Add the ice cubes and serve chilled.
6. Enjoy!

NUTRITION

- Calories: 155
- Fat: 14.6 g
- Fiber: 0.8 g
- Carbs: 8.6 g
- Protein: 4.6 g

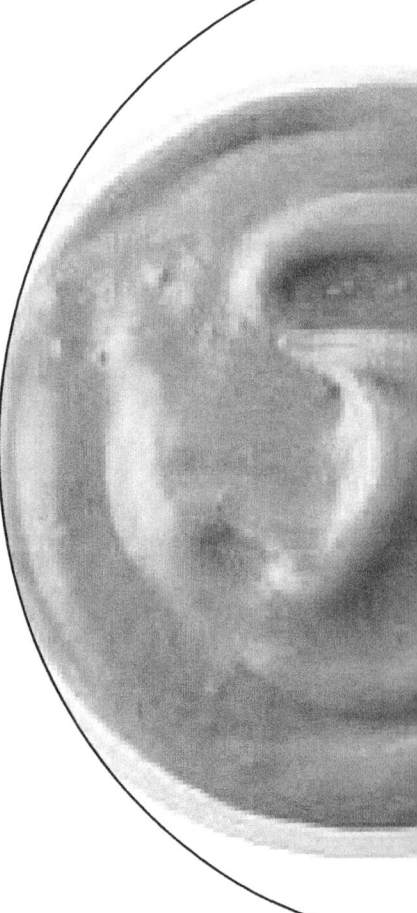

CHOCNUT SMOOTHIE

Preparation Time: 5 minutes
Cooking Time: 10 minutes
Servings: 2

INGREDIENTS

- 1 large cup of coconut milk, full fat
- ½ avocado, ripe
- 30 g of cacao powder
- 180 g of frozen cherries
- ¼ teaspoon of turmeric powder
- 230 ml cup of water
- Ice cubes

DIRECTIONS

1. Start by preparing all the ingredients together, then wash the avocado properly with water and coarsely chop it using a knife.
2. Add it to a blender, then stir in the cacao powder, roughly chopped cherries, and turmeric powder, and give it a whisk.
3. Add the water, coconut milk, and blend all the ingredients until it forms a smooth paste.
4. Pour it into a large glass and add some ice cubes to serve.
5. You can also refrigerate the smoothie for about 30 minutes before serving.
6. Enjoy!

NUTRITION

- Calories: 195
- Fat: 14.6 g
- Fiber: 0.8 g
- Carbs: 8.6 g
- Protein: 4.6 g

COCO STRAWBERRY SMOOTHIE

Preparation Time: 5 minutes
Cooking Time: 10 minutes
Servings: 2

INGREDIENTS

- 180 g of frozen strawberries
- 230 ml of coconut milk, unsweetened
- 2 tablespoons of almond butter
- 1 tablespoon of peanut butter
- 2 packets of stevia
- 1 teaspoon of chia seeds
- Crushed ice
- Mint leaves

DIRECTIONS

1. Start by preparing all the ingredients together, then wash the strawberries properly with water and coarsely chop it using a knife.
2. Add the strawberries to a blender, then stir in the almond butter, coconut milk, peanut butter, chia seeds, stevia drops and blend it using a hand blender.
3. Pour in a tall glass and add the crushed ice.
4. Garnish with mint leaves and serve.
5. Enjoy!

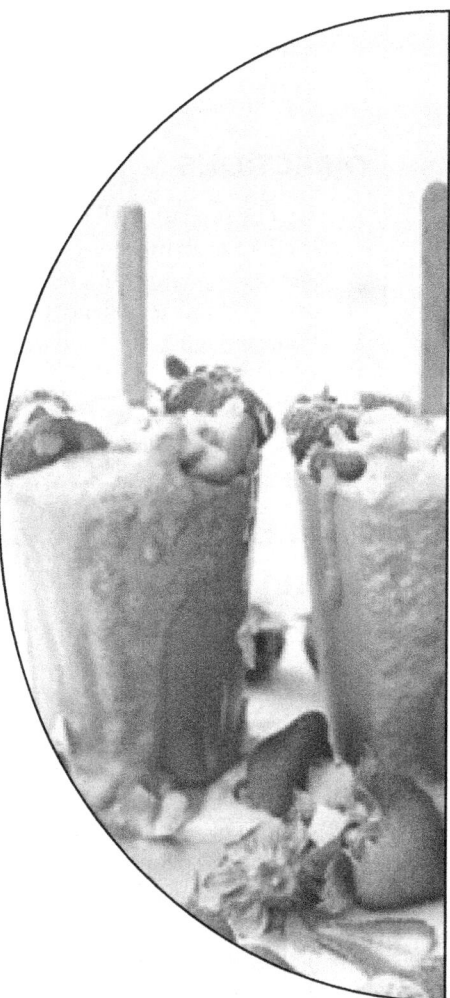

EGG SPINACH BERRIES SMOOTHIE

Preparation Time: 5 minutes
Cooking Time: 10 minutes
Servings: 2

INGREDIENTS

- 1 large egg
- 60 ml of coconut milk
- 180 g of berries
- 365 g of baby spinach, thawed
- ¼ avocado, sliced
- Crushed ice

DIRECTIONS

1. Start by preparing all the ingredients together, then wash the berries properly with water and coarsely chop it using a knife.
2. Wash the baby spinach and chop it up with the knife.
3. Add the chopped spinach, berries, and sliced avocado to the blender and whisk.
4. Add the coconut milk, crack an egg and whisk again until smooth.
5. Add the crushed ice to this smoothie and serve chilled.
6. Enjoy!

CREAMY DESSERT SMOOTHIE

Preparation Time: 5 minutes
Cooking Time: 10 minutes
Servings: 2

INGREDIENTS

- 175 ml cup of coconut milk
- 60 ml of sour cream
- 2 tablespoons of flaxseed meal
- 1 tablespoon of macadamia nut oil
- 20 drops of stevia
- ½ teaspoon of mango essence
- ¼ teaspoon of banana essence
- Crushed ice

DIRECTIONS

1. Start by preparing all the ingredients together, then add the flaxseed meal to some coconut milk in a bowl and let it soak up for 10 minutes.
2. Stir in the sour cream, macadamia oil, stevia, mango essence, banana essence, and mix. Add this to a blender and whisk until smooth.
3. Pour into tall glasses and add crushed ice to them.
4. Serve chilled.
5. Enjoy!

NUTRITION

- Calories: 187
- Fat: 14.6 g
- Fiber: 0.8 g
- Carbs: 8.6 g
- Protein: 4.6 g

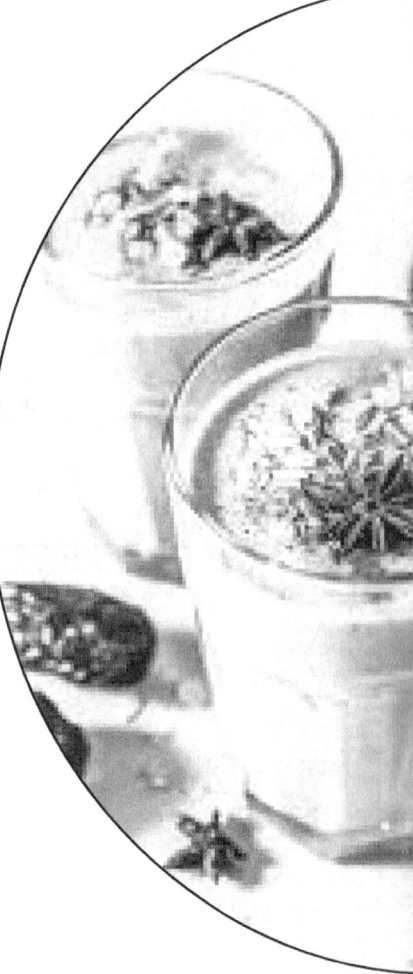

SWEET BUNS

Preparation Time: 40 minutes
Cooking Time: 30 minutes
Servings: 2

INGREDIENTS

- 1/3 cup of psyllium husks
- 1/2 cup of coconut flour
- 2 tablespoons of Swerve
- 4 eggs
- 1 teaspoon of baking powder
- 1/2 teaspoon of cinnamon
- 1/2 teaspoon of cloves; ground
- Some chocolate chips; unsweetened
- 1 cup of hot water
- A pinch of salt

DIRECTIONS

1. In a bowl, mix flour with psyllium husks, swerve, baking powder, salt, cinnamon, cloves, and chocolate chips and stir well.
2. Add water and eggs; stir well until you obtain a dough, shape 8 buns, and arrange them on a lined baking sheet.
3. Introduce in the oven at 350 ºF and bake for 30 minutes
4. Serve these buns with some almond milk, and enjoy!

NUTRITION

- Calories: 100
- Fat: 3 g
- Fiber: 3 g
- Carbs: 6 g
- Protein: 6 g

EASY MACAROONS

Preparation Time: 20 minutes
Cooking Time: 10 minutes
Servings: 2

INGREDIENTS

- 2 cup of coconut; shredded
- 1 teaspoon of vanilla extract
- 4 egg whites
- 2 tablespoons of stevia

DIRECTIONS

1. In a bowl, mix egg whites with stevia and beat using your mixer.
2. Add coconut and vanilla extract and stir.
3. Roll this mixture into small balls and place them on a lined baking sheet.
4. Introduce in the oven at 350 º F and bake for 10 minutes
5. Serve your macaroons cold.

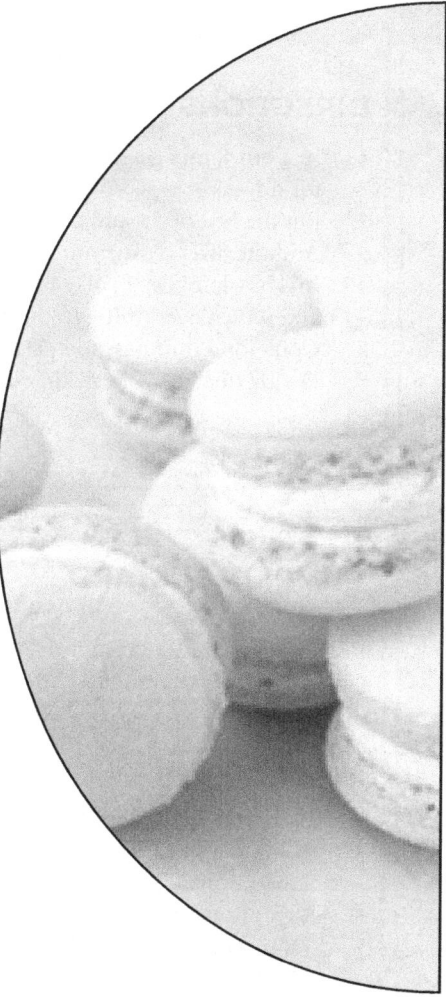

DELICIOUS CHOCOLATE TRUFFLES

Preparation Time: 16 minutes
Cooking Time: 10 minutes
Servings: 2

INGREDIENTS

- 1 cup of sugar-free chocolate chips
- 2 tablespoons of butter
- 2 teaspoons of brandy
- 2 tablespoons of Swerve
- 2/3 cup of heavy cream
- 1/4 teaspoon of vanilla extract
- Cocoa powder

DIRECTIONS

1. Put the heavy cream in a heatproof bowl, add swerve, butter, and chocolate chips; stir, introduce in your microwave and heat up for 1 minute.
2. Leave it aside for 5 minutes; stir well and mix with brandy and vanilla.
3. Stir again, leave aside in the fridge for a couple of hours.
4. Use a melon baller to shape your truffles, roll them in cocoa powder and serve them.

COCONUT PUDDING

Preparation Time: 20 minutes
Cooking Time: 10 minutes
Servings: 2

INGREDIENTS

- 1 2/3 cups of coconut milk
- 1/2 teaspoon of vanilla extract
- 3 egg yolks
- 1 tablespoon of gelatin
- 6 tablespoons of Swerve

DIRECTIONS

1. In a bowl, mix gelatin with 1-tablespoon of coconut milk; stir well and leave aside for now.
2. Put the rest of the milk into a pan and heat up over medium heat.
3. Add the Swerve; stir, and cook for 5 minutes.
4. In a bowl, mix egg yolks with the hot coconut milk and vanilla extract; stir well and return everything to the pan.
5. Cook for 4 minutes, add gelatin and stir well.
6. Divide this into 4 ramekins and keep your pudding in the fridge until you serve it.

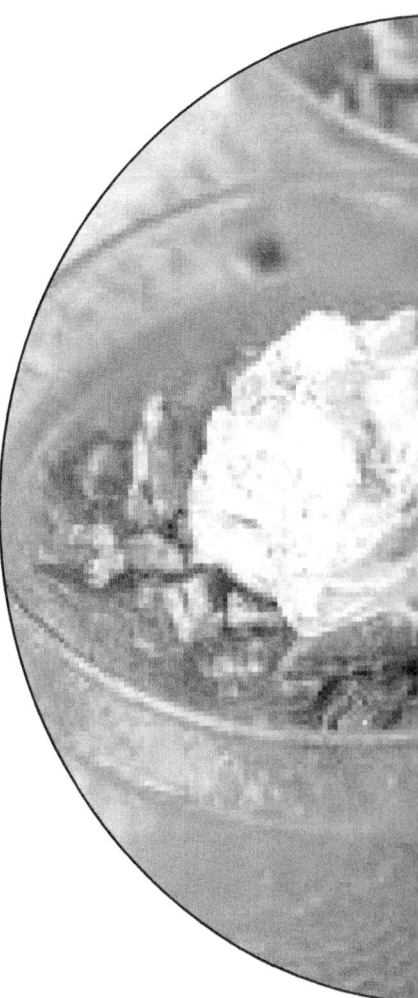

PUMPKIN CUSTARD

Preparation Time: 15 minutes
Cooking Time: 10 minutes
Servings: 2

INGREDIENTS

- 14 ounces of canned coconut milk
- 14 ounces of canned pumpkin puree
- 2 teaspoons of vanilla extract
- 8 scoops of stevia
- 3 tablespoons of Erythritol
- 1 tablespoon of gelatin
- 1/4 cup of warm water
- A pinch of salt
- 1 teaspoon of cinnamon powder
- 1 teaspoon of pumpkin pie spice

DIRECTIONS

1. In a pot, mix pumpkin puree with coconut milk, a pinch of salt, vanilla extract, cinnamon powder, stevia, Erythritol, and pumpkin pie spice; stir well and heat up for a couple of minutes
2. In a bowl, mix gelatin and water and stir.
3. Combine the 2 mixtures; stir well, divide custard into ramekins and leave aside to cool down.
4. Keep in the fridge until you serve it.

YUMMY ORANGE CAKE

Preparation Time: 30 minutes
Cooking Time: 20 minutes
Servings: 2

INGREDIENTS

- 1 orange; cut into quarters
- 1 teaspoon of vanilla extract
- 1 teaspoon of baking powder
- 4 ounces of cream cheese
- 4 ounces of coconut yogurt
- 9 ounces of almond meal
- 2 tablespoons of orange zest
- 2 ounces of stevia
- 6 eggs
- 4 tablespoons of Swerve
- A pinch of salt

DIRECTIONS

1. In your food processor, pulse the orange very well.
2. Add the almond meal, swerve, eggs, baking powder, vanilla extract, and a pinch of salt, and pulse well again.
3. Transfer this into 2 springform pans, introduce in the oven at 350 °F and bake for 20 minutes.
4. Meanwhile, in a bowl, mix the cream cheese with orange zest, coconut yogurt, stevia, and stir well.
5. Place one cake layer on a plate, add half of the cream cheese mix, add the other cake layer, and top with the rest of the cream cheese mix.
6. Spread it well, slice and serve.

NUTRITION

- Calories: 200
- Fat: 13 g
- Fiber: 2 g
- Carbs: 5 g
- Protein: 8 g

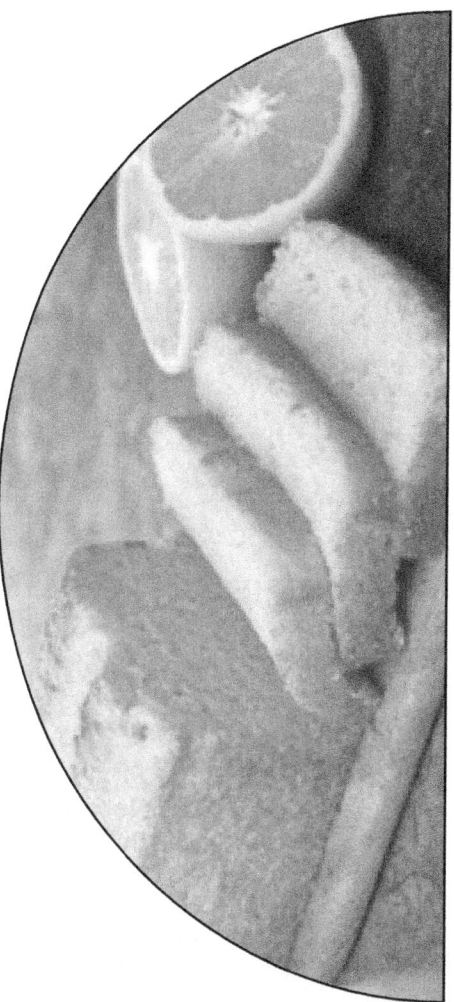

MUG CAKE

Preparation Time: 5 minutes
Cooking Time: 10 minutes
Servings: 2

INGREDIENTS

- 4 tablespoons of almond meal
- 1 tablespoon of coconut flour
- 2 tablespoon of ghee
- 1 teaspoon of stevia
- 1/4 teaspoon of vanilla extract
- 1/2 teaspoon of baking powder
- 1 tablespoon of cocoa powder; unsweetened
- 1 egg

DIRECTIONS

1. Put the ghee in a mug and introduce it in the microwave for a couple of seconds.
2. Add cocoa powder, stevia, egg, baking powder, vanilla, and coconut flour and stir well.
3. Add almond meal as well; stir again, introduce in the microwave and cook for 2 minutes.
4. Serve your mug cake with berries on top.

NUTRITION

- Calories: 450
- Fat: 34 g
- Fiber: 7 g
- Carbs: 10 g
- Protein: 20 g

MARSHMALLOWS

Preparation Time: 13 minutes
Cooking Time: 10 minutes
Servings: 2

INGREDIENTS

- 12 scoops of stevia
- 2 tablespoons of gelatin
- ¾ cup of Erythritol
- 1/2 cup of cold water
- 2 teaspoons of vanilla extract
- 1/2 cup of hot water

DIRECTIONS

1. In a bowl, mix the gelatin with cold water; stir and leave aside for 5 minutes
2. Put hot water in a pan, add Erythritol and stevia and stir well.
3. Combine this with the gelatin mix, add vanilla extract and stir everything well.
4. Beat this using a mixer and pour it into a baking pan.
5. Leave aside in the fridge until it sets, then cut into pieces and serve.

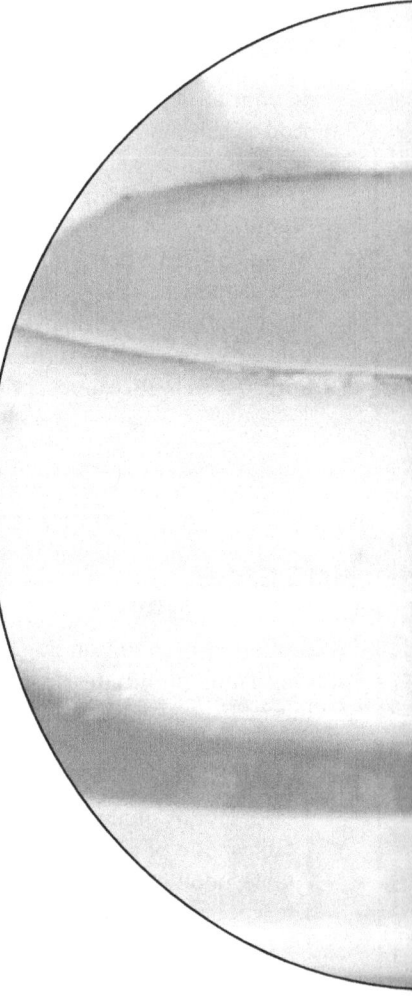

CARAMEL CUSTARD

Preparation Time: 40 minutes
Cooking Time: 30 minutes
Servings: 2

INGREDIENTS

- 1½ teaspoons of caramel extract
- 1½ tablespoons of Swerve
- 2 ounces of cream cheese
- 2 eggs
- 1 cup of water

For the caramel sauce:
- 1/4 teaspoon of caramel extract
- 2 tablespoons of Swerve
- 2 tablespoons of ghee

DIRECTIONS

1. In your blender, mix the cream cheese with water, 1½ tablespoons of swerve, 1½ teaspoons of caramel extract, eggs, and blend well.
2. Pour this into 2 greased ramekins, introduce in the oven at 350 ºF and bake for 30 minutes.
3. Meanwhile, put the ghee in a pot and heat up over medium heat; add 1/4 teaspoon of caramel extract and 2 tablespoons of Swerve; stir well and cook until everything melts.
4. Pour this over caramel custard, leave everything to cool down and serve.

CHOCOLATE SHAKE

Preparation Time: 10 minutes
Cooking Time: 5 minutes
Servings: 2

INGREDIENTS

- 2 cups of heavy cream, whipped
- 1 tablespoon of cocoa powder
- 1 tablespoon of peanut butter
- ½ cup of coconut milk
- 2 tablespoons of Erythritol
- ½ teaspoon of vanilla extract

DIRECTIONS

1. Mix up the coconut milk and whipped heavy cream.
2. Add the cocoa powder and mix it with the help of the hand mixer.
3. When the liquid is homogenous, add peanut butter, vanilla extract, and Erythritol.
4. Whisk it well.
5. Pour the chocolate shake into the serving glasses.

NUTRITION
- Calories: 304
- Fat: 31.5 g
- Fiber: 1.3 g
- Carbs: 4.9 g
- Protein: 3.2 g

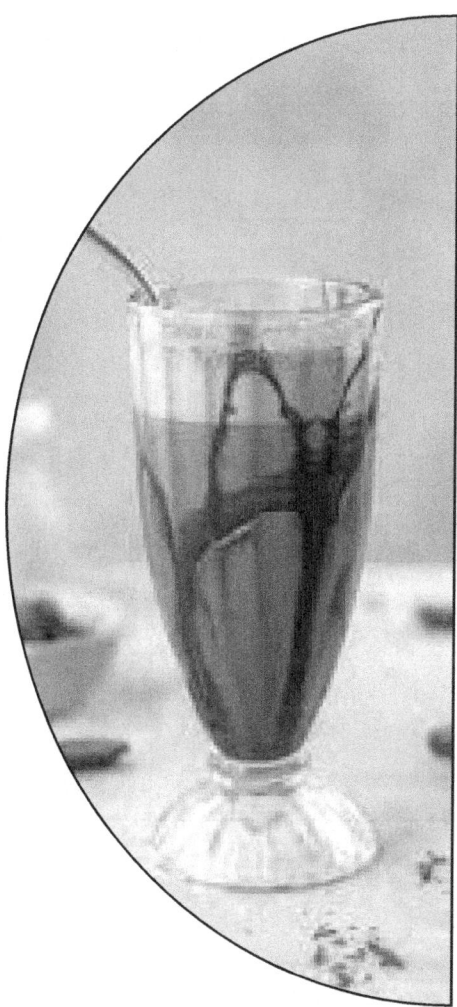

SMOOTHIE BOWL

Preparation Time: 7 minutes
Cooking Time: 0 minutes
Servings: 2

INGREDIENTS

- 1 teaspoon of pumpkin seeds
- 1 teaspoon of sunflower seeds
- ½ cup of blackberries
- 1 cup of almond milk
- ¼ cup of coconut cream
- 2 tablespoons of Erythritol
- 1 tablespoon of Protein powder
- ½ teaspoon of cocoa powder

DIRECTIONS

1. Blend the almond milk, coconut cream, blackberries, Erythritol, and protein powder.
2. When the mixture is smooth, add cocoa powder and pulse it for 30 seconds more.
3. Pour the liquid into the small serving bowls.
4. Sprinkle the smoothie with pumpkin seeds and sunflower seeds.

NUTRITION

- Calories: 346
- Fat: 11.5 g
- Fiber: 3.4 g
- Carbs: 11.5 g
- Protein: 5.6 g

CHAPTER 10.
EXTRA RECIPES

CHEESY HAM SOUFFLÉ

Preparation Time: 30 minutes
Cooking Time: 20 minutes
Servings: 2

INGREDIENTS

- 1 cup of cheddar cheese, shredded
- 6 large eggs
- Salt and black pepper, to taste
- 6 ounces of ham, diced

DIRECTIONS

1. Preheat the oven to 375 ºF and lightly grease the ramekins.
2. Whisk the ham with the rest of the ingredients in a bowl.
3. Mix well and pour the mixture into the ramekins.
4. Transfer to the oven and bake for about 20 minutes.
5. Remove from the oven and slightly cool before serving.

NUTRITION

- Calories: 342
- Total Fat: 26 g
- Saturated Fat: 13 g
- Cholesterol: 353 mg
- Sodium: 841 mg
- Total Carbohydrates: 3 g
- Dietary Fiber: 0.6 g
- Total Sugars: 0.8 g
- Protein: 23.8 g

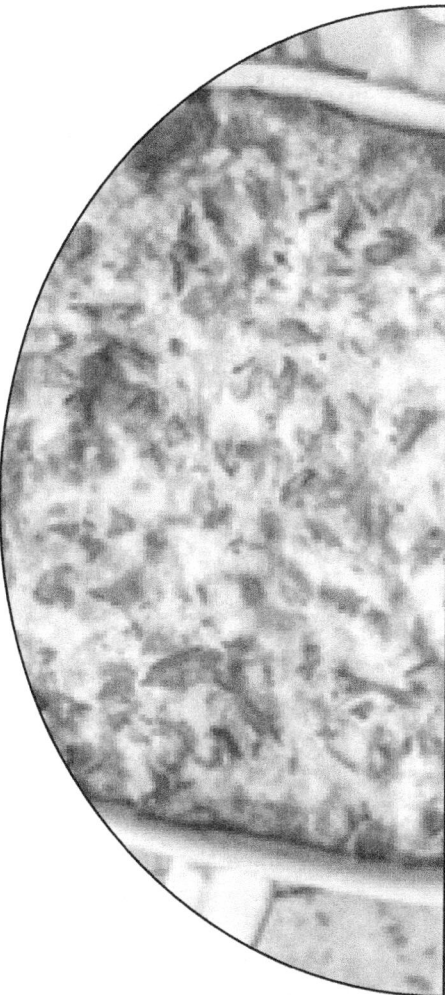

MUSHROOM AND CHEESE SCRAMBLED EGGS

Preparation Time: 20 minutes
Cooking Time: 15 minutes
Servings: 2

INGREDIENTS

- 8 eggs
- 4 tablespoons of butter
- 4 tablespoons of parmesan cheese, shredded
- 1 cup of fresh mushrooms, finely chopped
- Salt and black pepper, to taste

DIRECTIONS

1. Whisk the eggs with salt and black pepper in a bowl until well combined.
2. Heat the butter in a nonstick pan and stir in the whisked eggs.
3. Cook for about 4 minutes and add mushrooms and parmesan cheese.
4. Cook for about 6 minutes, occasionally stirring and dish out to serve.

NUTRITION

- Calories: 265
- Total Fat: 22.6 g
- Saturated Fat: 11.5 g
- Cholesterol: 365 mg
- Sodium: 304 mg
- Total Carbohydrates: 1.7 g
- Dietary Fiber: 0.2 g
- Total Sugars: 1 g
- Protein: 15.1 g

RED PEPPER FRITTATA

Preparation Time: 15 minutes
Cooking Time: 10 minutes
Servings: 2

INGREDIENTS

- 6 large eggs
- 2 red peppers, chopped
- Salt and black pepper, to taste
- 1¼ cups of mozzarella cheese, shredded
- 3 tablespoons of olive oil

DIRECTIONS

1. Whisk the eggs in a medium bowl and add red peppers, mozzarella cheese, salt and black pepper.
2. Heat the olive oil over medium-high heat in an ovenproof skillet and pour in the egg mixture.
3. Lift the mixture with a spatula to let the eggs run under.
4. Cook for about 5 minutes, stirring well and dish out onto a platter to serve.

NUTRITION

- Calories: 308
- Total Fat: 26.2 g
- Saturated Fat: 6.4 g
- Cholesterol: 378 mg
- Sodium: 214 mg
- Total Carbohydrates: 3.9 g
- Dietary Fiber: 0.5 g
- Total Sugars: 2.4 g
- Protein: 16.5 g

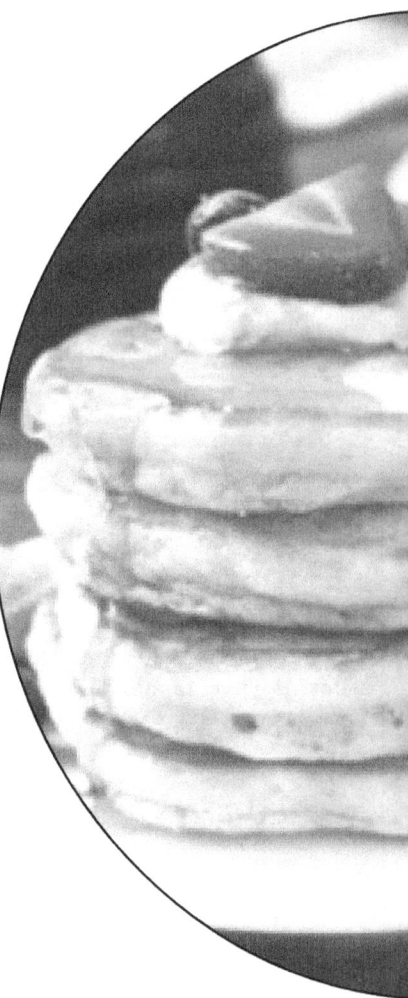

CREAM CHEESE PANCAKES

Preparation Time: 25 minutes
Cooking Time: 15 minutes
Servings: 2

INGREDIENTS

- ½ cup of almond flour
- 2 scoops of Stevia
- ½ teaspoon of cinnamon
- 2 eggs
- 2 oz. of cream cheese

DIRECTIONS

1. Put all the ingredients in a blender and blend until smooth.
2. Dish out the mixture to a medium bowl and set aside.
3. Heat the butter in a skillet over medium heat and add one-quarter of the mixture.
4. Spread the mixture and cook for about 4 minutes on both sides until golden brown.
5. Repeat with the rest of the mixture in batches and serve warm.

NUTRITION

- Calories: 166
- Total Fat: 13.8 g
- Saturated Fat: 4.3 g
- Cholesterol: 97 mg
- Sodium: 78 mg
- Total Carbohydrates: 3.8 g
- Dietary Fiber: 1.7 g
- Total Sugars: 0.2 g
- Protein: 6.9 g

SPICY CHORIZO BAKED EGGS

Preparation Time: 40 minutes
Cooking Time: 30 minutes
Servings: 2

INGREDIENTS

- 5 large eggs
- 3 ounces of ground chorizo sausage
- ¾ cup of pepper jack cheese, shredded
- Salt and paprika, to taste
- 1 small avocado, chopped

DIRECTIONS

1. Preheat the oven to 400 °F.
2. Heat a nonstick oven-safe skillet and add chorizo.
3. Cook for about 8 minutes and dish into a bowl.
4. Break the eggs in the skillet and season with salt and paprika.
5. Add the cooked chorizo and avocado and cook for about 2 minutes.
6. Top with pepper jack cheese and transfer to the oven.
7. Bake for about 20 minutes and remove from the oven to serve.

NUTRITION

- Calories: 334
- Total Fat: 28.3 g
- Saturated Fat: 10.3 g
- Cholesterol: 269 mg
- Sodium: 400 mg
- Total Carbohydrates: 5.7 g
- Dietary Fiber: 3.6 g
- Total Sugars: 0.8 g
- Protein: 16.9 g

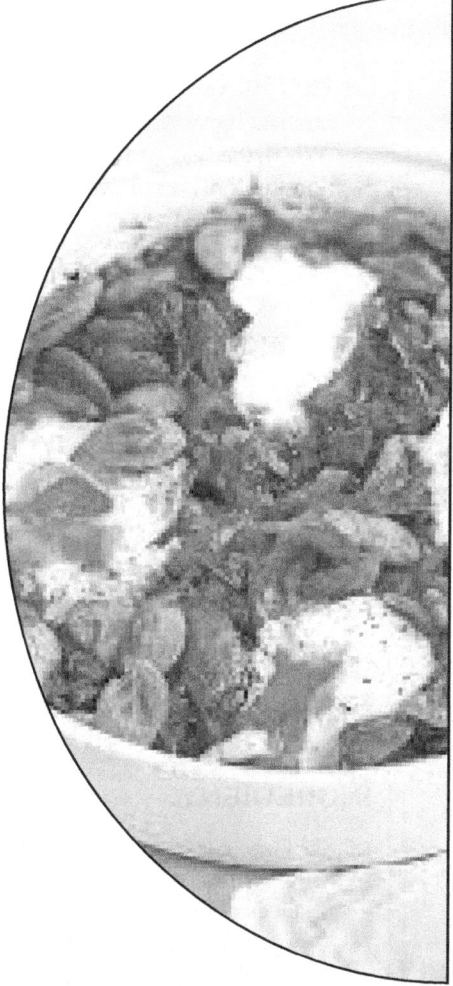

CHEESY TACO PIE

Preparation Time: 15 minutes
Cooking Time: 45 minutes
Servings: 2

INGREDIENTS

- 1 tablespoon of garlic powder
- 1 pound of ground beef
- Salt and chili powder, to taste
- 1 cup of cheddar cheese, shredded

DIRECTIONS

1. Preheat the oven to 350 °F and lightly grease a pie plate.
2. Heat a large nonstick skillet and add beef, garlic powder, salt and chili powder.
3. Cook for about 6 minutes over medium-low heat and transfer to the pie plate.
4. Top with cheddar cheese and transfer to the oven.
5. Bake for about 30 minutes and remove from the oven to serve hot.

NUTRITION

- Calories: 294
- Total Fat: 16 g
- Saturated Fat: 7.3 g
- Cholesterol: 273 mg
- Sodium: 241 mg
- Total Carbohydrates: 1.9 g
- Dietary Fiber: 0.3 g
- Total Sugars: 0.9 g
- Protein: 34.2 g

SAUSAGE EGG CASSEROLE

Preparation Time: 40 minutes
Cooking Time: 30 minutes
Servings: 2

INGREDIENTS

- 1 cup of almond milk, unsweetened
- 6 large eggs
- Salt and black pepper, to taste
- 2 cups of cheddar cheese, shredded
- 1 pound of ground pork sausage, cooked

DIRECTIONS

1. Preheat the oven to 350 °F and lightly grease a casserole dish.
2. Whisk the eggs with almond milk, salt and black pepper in a bowl.
3. Put the cooked sausages in the casserole dish and top with the egg mixture and cheddar cheese.
4. Transfer to the oven and bake for about 30 minutes.
5. Remove from the oven and serve hot.

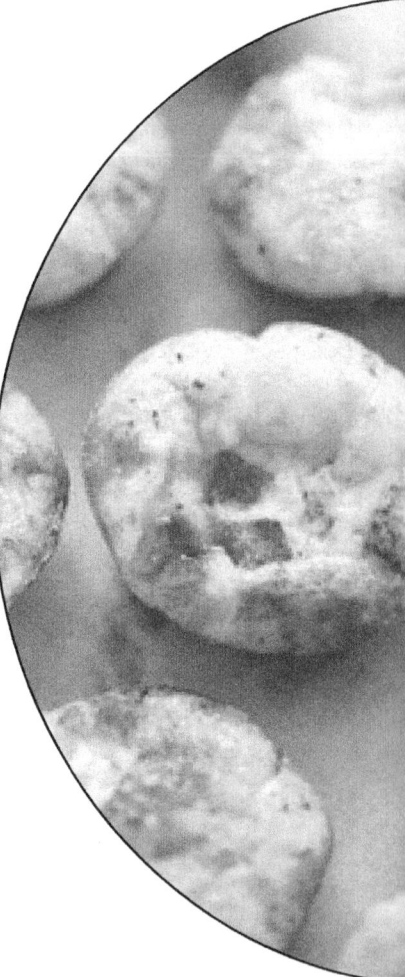

EGG BITES

Preparation Time: 25 minutes
Cooking Time: 15 minutes
Servings: 6

INGREDIENTS

- 12 large eggs
- 1 -8 ounces of package of cream cheese, softened
- 8 slices of bacon, cooked and crumbled
- 1 cup of gruyere cheese, shredded
- Salt and paprika, to taste

DIRECTIONS

1. Put the eggs, cream cheese, salt and paprika in a blender and blend until smooth.
2. Grease 8 egg poaching cups lightly with cooking spray and put half the gruyere cheese, bacon and egg mixture in them.
3. Put the cups in a large saucepan with boiling water and cover the lid.
4. Lower the heat and cook for about 10 minutes.
5. Dish out the eggs into a serving dish and slice to serve.

CHORIZO AND EGGS

Preparation Time: 20 minutes
Cooking Time: 15 minutes
Servings: 2

INGREDIENTS

- ½ small yellow onion, chopped
- 1 teaspoon of olive oil
- 2 -3 ounces of chorizo sausage
- Salt and black pepper, to taste
- 4 eggs

DIRECTIONS

1. Open the sausage casings and dish the meat into a bowl.
2. Heat the olive oil over medium-high heat in a large skillet and add onions.
3. Sauté for about 3 minutes and stir in the chorizo sausage.
4. Cook for about 4 minutes and add eggs, salt and black pepper.
5. Whisk well and cook for about 3 minutes.
6. Dish into a bowl and serve warm.

NUTRITION

- Calories: 270
- Total Fat: 21.8 g
- Saturated Fat: 7.6 g
- Cholesterol: 201 mg
- Sodium: 587 mg
- Total Carbohydrates: 2 g
- Dietary Fiber: 0.2 g
- Total Sugars: 0.7 g
- Protein: 15.9 g

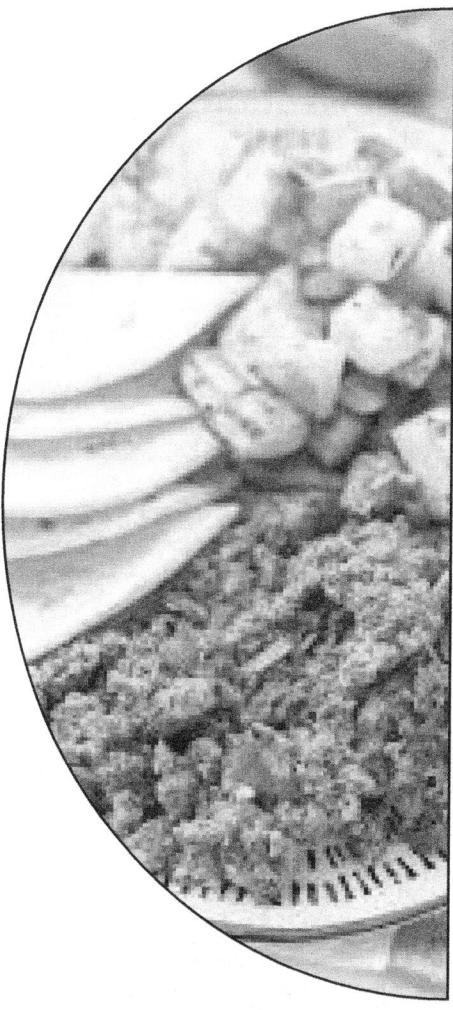

EGG, BACON, AND CHEESE CUPS

Preparation Time: 30 minutes
Cooking Time: 15 minutes
Servings: 2

INGREDIENTS

- ¼ cup of frozen spinach, thawed and drained
- 6 large eggs
- 6 strips of bacon
- Salt and black pepper, to taste
- ¼ cup of sharp cheddar cheese

DIRECTIONS

1. Preheat the oven to 400 ºF and grease 6 muffin cups.
2. Whisk the eggs, spinach, salt and black pepper in a bowl.
3. Put the bacon slices in the muffin cups and pour in the egg spinach mixture.
4. Top with the sharp cheddar cheese and transfer to the oven.
5. Bake for 15 minutes and remove from the oven to serve warm.

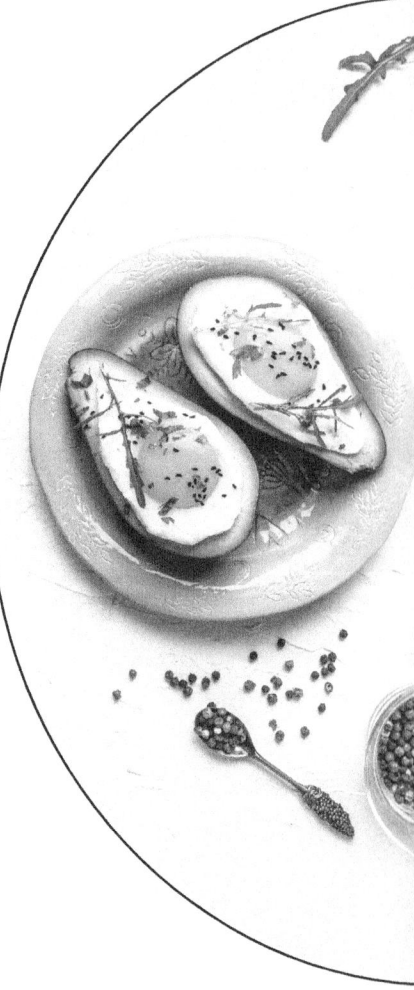

NUTRITION

- Calories: 270
- Total Fat: 21.8 g
- Saturated Fat: 7.6 g
- Cholesterol: 201 mg
- Sodium: 587 mg
- Total Carbohydrates: 2 g
- Dietary Fiber: 0.2 g
- Total Sugars: 0.7 g
- Protein: 15.9 g

EGG IN THE AVOCADO

Preparation Time: 25 minutes
Cooking Time: 15 minutes
Servings: 2

INGREDIENTS

- 3 medium avocados, cut in half, pitted, skin on
- 1 teaspoon of garlic powder
- ¼ cup of parmesan cheese, grated
- 6 medium eggs
- Sea salt and black pepper, to taste

DIRECTIONS

1. Preheat the oven to 350 ºF and grease 6 muffin tins.
2. Put the avocado half in each muffin tin and season with garlic powder, sea salt, and black pepper.
3. Break 1 egg into each avocado and top with the parmesan cheese.
4. Transfer into the oven and bake for about 15 minutes.
5. Remove from the oven and serve warm.

NUTRITION

- Calories: 194
- Total Fat: 14.5 g
- Saturated Fat: 5.2 g
- Cholesterol: 212 mg
- Sodium: 539 mg
- Total Carbohydrates: 0.8 g
- Dietary Fiber: 0 g
- Total Sugars: 0.4 g
- Protein: 14.5 g
-

STEAK AND EGGS

Preparation Time: 25 minutes
Cooking Time: 15 minutes
Servings: 2

INGREDIENTS

- 6 eggs
- 2 tablespoons of butter
- 8 oz. of sirloin steak
- Salt and black pepper, to taste
- ½ avocado, sliced

DIRECTIONS

1. Heat the butter in a pan on medium heat and fry the eggs.
2. Season with salt and black pepper and dish out onto a plate.
3. Cook the sirloin steak in another pan until desired doneness and slice into bite-sized strips.
4. Season with salt and black pepper and dish out alongside the eggs.
5. Put the avocados with the eggs and steaks and serve.

NUTRITION

- Calories: 302
- Total Fat: 20.8 g
- Saturated Fat: 8.1 g
- Cholesterol: 311 mg
- Sodium: 172 mg
- Total Carbohydrates: 2.7 g
- Dietary Fiber: 1.7 g
- Total Sugars: 0.6 g
- Protein: 26 g

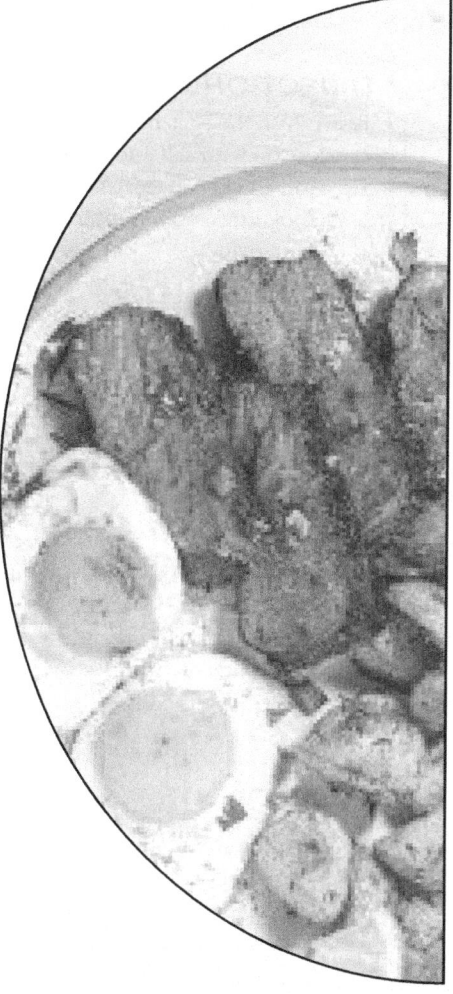

BUTTER COFFEE

Preparation Time: 20 minutes
Cooking Time: 10 minutes
Servings: 2

INGREDIENTS

- ½ cup of coconut milk
- ½ cup of water
- 2 tablespoons of coffee
- 1 tablespoon of coconut oil
- 1 tablespoon grass-fed butter

DIRECTIONS

1. Heat the water in a saucepan and add coffee.
2. Simmer for about 3 minutes and add coconut milk.
3. Simmer for another 3 minutes and allow to cool down.
4. Transfer to a blender along with coconut oil and butter.
5. Pour into a mug and serve immediately.

NUTRITION

- Calories: 111
- Total Fat: 11.9 g
- Saturated Fat: 10.3 g
- Cholesterol: 4 mg
- Sodium: 18 mg
- Total Carbohydrates: 1.7 g
- Dietary Fiber: 0.7 g
- Total Sugars: 1 g
- Protein: 0.7 g

CALIFORNIA CHICKEN OMELET

Preparation Time: 20 minutes
Cooking Time: 15 minutes
Servings: 2

INGREDIENTS

- 2 bacon slices, cooked and chopped
- 2 eggs
- 1 oz. of deli cut chicken
- 3 tablespoons of avocado mayonnaise
- 1 Campari tomato

DIRECTIONS

1. Whisk the eggs in a bowl and pour into a nonstick pan.
2. Season with salt and black pepper and cook for about 5 minutes.
3. Add chicken, bacon, tomato and avocado mayonnaise and cover with lid.
4. Cook for 5 more minutes on medium-low heat and dish out to serve hot.

NUTRITION

- Calories: 208
- Total Fat: 15 g
- Saturated Fat: 4.5 g
- Cholesterol: 189 mg
- Sodium: 658 mg
- Total Carbohydrates: 3 g
- Dietary Fiber: 1.1 g
- Total Sugars: 0.9 g
- Protein: 15.3 g

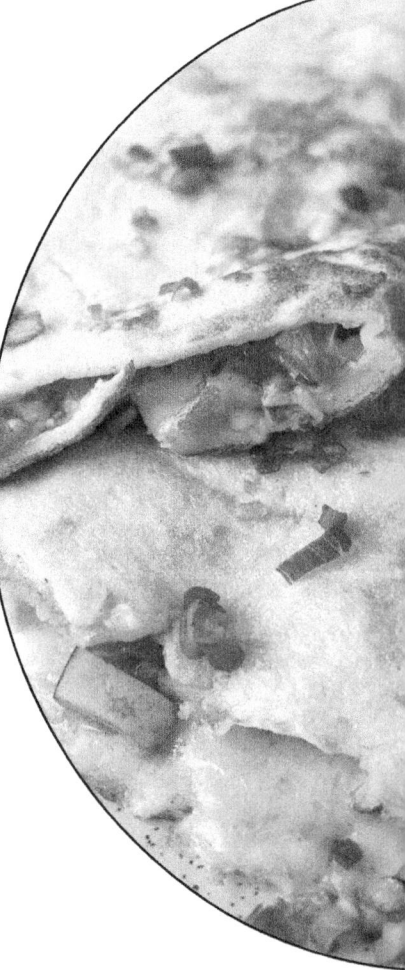

EGGS OOPSIE ROLLS

Preparation Time: 25 minutes
Cooking Time: 40 minutes
Servings: 2

INGREDIENTS

- 3 oz. of cream cheese
- 3 large eggs, separated
- 1/8 teaspoon of cream of tartar
- 1 scoop of stevia
- 1/8 teaspoon of salt

DIRECTIONS

1. Preheat the oven to 300 °F and line a cookie sheet with parchment paper.
2. Beat the egg whites with cream of tartar until soft peaks form.
3. Mix the egg yolks, salt, stevia, and cream cheese in a bowl.
4. Combine the egg yolk and egg white mixtures and spoon them onto the cookie sheet.
5. Transfer to the oven and bake for about 40 minutes.
6. Remove from the oven and serve warm.

NUTRITION

- Calories: 171
- Total Fat: 14.9 g
- Saturated Fat: 7.8 g
- Cholesterol: 217 mg
- Sodium: 251 mg
- Total Carbohydrates: 1.2 g
- Dietary Fiber: 0 g
- Total Sugars: 0.5 g
- Protein: 8.4 g

SHAKSHUKA

Preparation Time: 25 minutes
Cooking Time: 15 minutes
Servings: 2

INGREDIENTS

- 1 chili pepper, chopped
- 1 cup of marinara sauce
- 4 eggs
- Salt and black pepper, to taste
- 1 oz. of feta cheese

DIRECTIONS

1. Preheat the oven to 390 °F.
2. Heat a small ovenproof skillet on medium heat and add marinara sauce and chili pepper.
3. Cook for about 5 minutes and stir in the eggs.
4. Season with salt and black pepper and top with feta cheese.
5. Transfer into the oven and bake for about 15 minutes.
6. Remove from the oven and serve hot Shakshuka.

NUTRITION

- Calories: 273
- Total Fat: 15.1 g
- Saturated Fat: 5.7 g
- Cholesterol: 342 mg
- Sodium: 794 mg
- Total Carbohydrates: 18.7 g
- Dietary Fiber: 3.3 g
- Total Sugars: 12.4 g
- Protein: 15.4 g

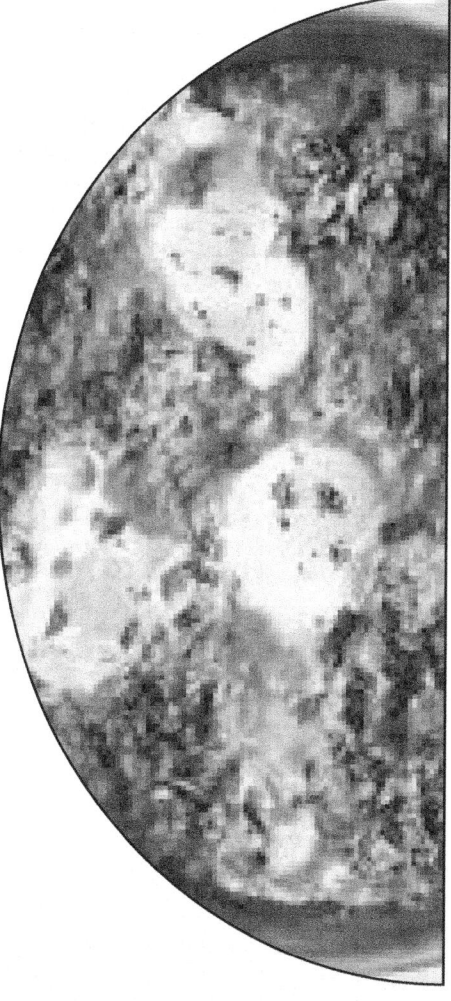

ROOIBOS TEA LATTE

Preparation Time: 20 minutes
Cooking Time: 15 minutes
Servings: 2

INGREDIENTS

- 2 bags of rooibos tea
- 1 cup of water
- 1 tablespoon of grass fed butter
- 1 scoop of collagen peptides
- ¼ cup of full fat canned coconut milk

DIRECTIONS

1. Put the tea bags in boiling water and steep for about 5 minutes.
2. Discard the tea bags and stir in butter and coconut milk.
3. Pour this mixture into a blender and blend until smooth.
4. Add the collagen to the blender and blend at low speed until incorporated.
5. Pour into a mug to serve hot or chilled as desired.

NUTRITION

- Calories: 283
- Total Fat: 23.5 g
- Saturated Fat: 18.3 g
- Cholesterol: 31 mg
- Sodium: 21 mg
- Total Carbohydrates: 3.4 g
- Dietary Fiber: 0 g
- Total Sugars: 2.4 g
- Protein: 15 g

FETA AND PESTO OMELET

Preparation Time: 10 minutes
Cooking Time: 15 minutes
Servings: 2

INGREDIENTS

- 3 eggs
- 2 tablespoons of butter
- 1 oz. of feta cheese
- Salt and black pepper, to taste
- 1 tablespoon of pesto

DIRECTIONS

1. Heat the butter in a pan and allow it to melt.
2. Whisk the eggs in a bowl and pour into the pan.
3. Cook for about 3 minutes until done, and add feta cheese and pesto.
4. Season with salt and black pepper and fold it over.
5. Cook for another 5 minutes until the feta cheese is melted and dish out onto a platter to serve.

NUTRITION

- Calories: 178
- Total Fat: 16.2 g
- Saturated Fat: 8.1 g
- Cholesterol: 194 mg
- Sodium: 253 mg
- Total Carbohydrates: 1.1 g
- Dietary Fiber: 0.1 g
- Total Sugars: 1.1 g
- Protein: 7.5 g

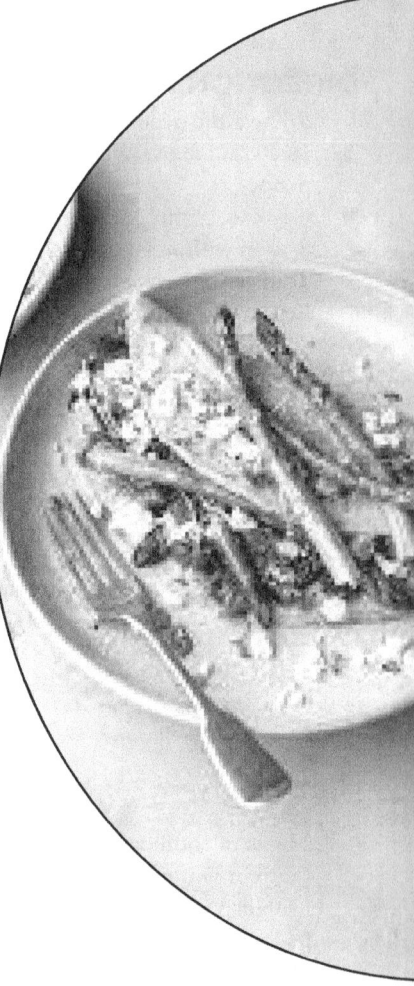

EGGS BENEDICT

Preparation Time: 25 minutes
Cooking Time: 15 minutes
Servings: 2

INGREDIENTS

- 4 Oopsie rolls
- 4 eggs
- 4 Canadian bacon slices, cooked and crisped
- 1 tablespoon of white vinegar
- 1 teaspoon of chives

DIRECTIONS

1. Boil water with vinegar and create a whirlpool in it with a wooden spoon.
2. Break an egg in a cup and place in the boiling water for about 3 minutes.
3. Repeat with the rest of the eggs and dish out onto a platter.
4. Place Oopsie rolls on the plates and top with bacon slices.
5. Put the poached eggs onto bacon slices and garnish with chives to serve.

NUTRITION

- Calories: 190
- Total Fat: 13.5 g
- Saturated Fat: 5.8 g
- Cholesterol: 275 mg
- Sodium: 587 mg
- Total Carbohydrates: 1.5 g
- Dietary Fiber: 0 g
- Total Sugars: 0.6 g
- Protein: 15.3 g

EGG CLOUDS

Preparation Time: 25 minutes
Cooking Time: 15 minutes
Servings: 2

INGREDIENTS

- 6 strips of bacon
- ¼ teaspoon of cayenne pepper
- 2 eggs, separated
- Salt and black pepper, to taste
- ½ teaspoon of garlic powder

DIRECTIONS

1. Preheat oven to 350 °F and grease a baking sheet lightly.
2. Whisk the egg whites in a bowl until fluffy and add garlic powder and salt.
3. Make 2 bacon weaves and spoon the egg white mixture on to it to form a cloud.
4. Make a hole in the egg cloud and put the egg yolks in it.
5. Season with cayenne pepper and black pepper and transfer to the oven.
6. Bake for about 10 minutes and dish out on a platter to serve.

NUTRITION

- Calories: 374
- Total Fat: 28.2 g
- Saturated Fat: 9.2 g
- Cholesterol: 226 mg
- Sodium: 379 mg
- Total Carbohydrates: 1.8 g
- Dietary Fiber: 0.1 g
- Total Sugars: 0.5 g
- Protein: 26.8 g

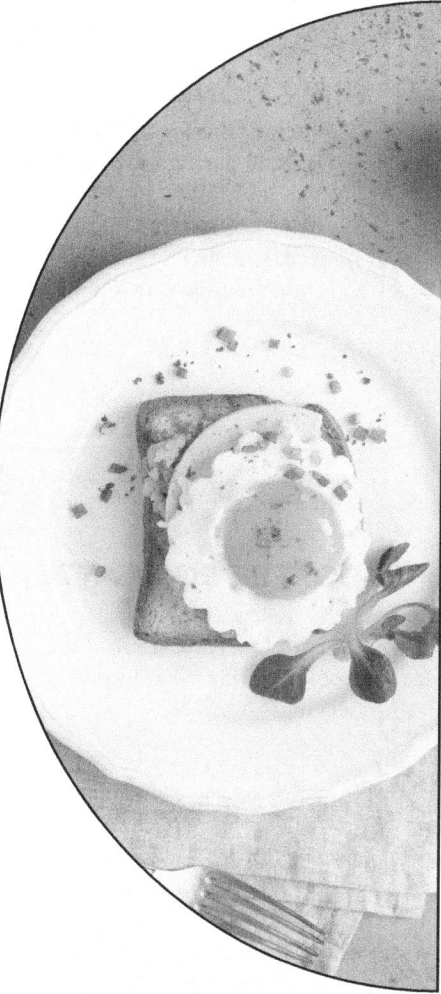

SPICY SHRIMP OMELET

Preparation Time: 15 minutes
Cooking Time: 15 minutes
Servings: 2

INGREDIENTS

- 6 eggs
- 10 large shrimp, boiled
- 4 grape tomatoes
- Sriracha salt and cayenne pepper, to taste
- 1 handful of spinach

DIRECTIONS

1. Whisk the eggs with all other ingredients in a bowl.
2. Heat a nonstick pan and pour the mixture into it.
3. Cook for about 5 minutes on medium-low heat and flip the side.
4. Cook for another 5 minutes and dish out onto a platter to serve.

NUTRITION

- Calories: 90
- Total Fat: 4.7 g
- Saturated Fat: 1.4 g
- Cholesterol: 183 mg
- Sodium: 93 mg
- Total Carbohydrates: 3.9 g
- Dietary Fiber: 1.1 g
- Total Sugars: 2.5 g
- Protein: 8.5 g

EGG PIZZA CRUST

Preparation Time: 25 minutes
Cooking Time: 15 minutes
Servings: 2

INGREDIENTS

- 4 eggs
- 2 tablespoons of coconut flour
- 2 cups of cauliflower, grated
- ½ teaspoon of salt
- 1 tablespoon of psyllium husk powder

DIRECTIONS

1. Preheat the oven to 360 ºF and lightly grease a pizza tray.
2. Mix all the ingredients in a bowl until well combined and set it aside for about 10 minutes.
3. Pour this mixture into the pizza tray and place it in the oven.
4. Bake for about 15 minutes until golden brown and remove from the oven.
5. Add your favorite toppings and serve.

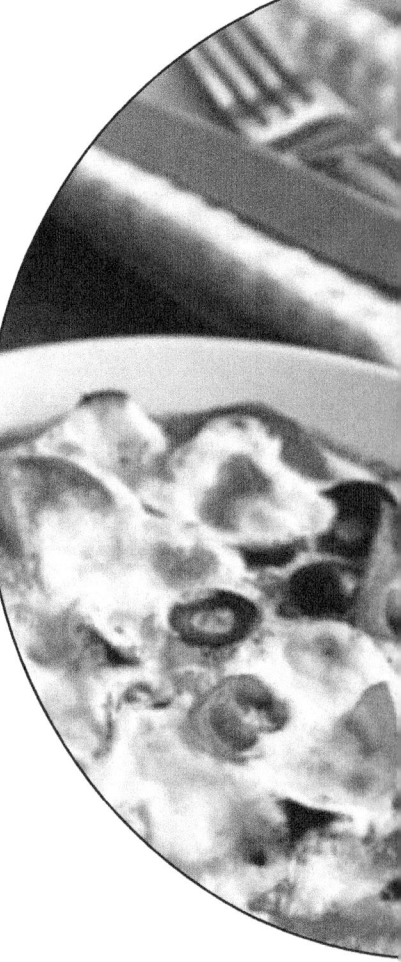

COFFEE EGG LATTE

Preparation Time: 15 minutes
Cooking Time: 5 minutes
Servings: 2

INGREDIENTS

- 8 ounces of black coffee
- 2 tablespoons of grass-fed butter
- 2 pasture-raised eggs
- 1 scoop of vanilla collagen protein
- ¼ teaspoon of Ceylon cinnamon

DIRECTIONS

1. Put the eggs, butter and coffee in a blender.
2. Blend until smooth and stir in the collagen protein.
3. Blend on low and pour into 2 mugs.
4. Sprinkle with cinnamon and serve hot or chilled as desired.

BUTTERY EGG WAFFLES

Preparation Time: 30 minutes
Cooking Time: 15 minutes
Servings: 2

INGREDIENTS

- 4 tablespoons of coconut flour
- 5 eggs, whites separated
- 4 scoops of Stevia
- 1 teaspoon of baking powder
- ½ cup of butter, melted

DIRECTIONS

1. Mix the coconut flour, egg yolks, Stevia and baking powder in a bowl.
2. Add the butter and mix well to form a smooth batter.
3. Whisk the egg whites in another bowl until fluffy and pour into the flour mixture.
4. Put this mixture into a waffle maker and cook until golden in color.
5. Dish out on plates to serve.

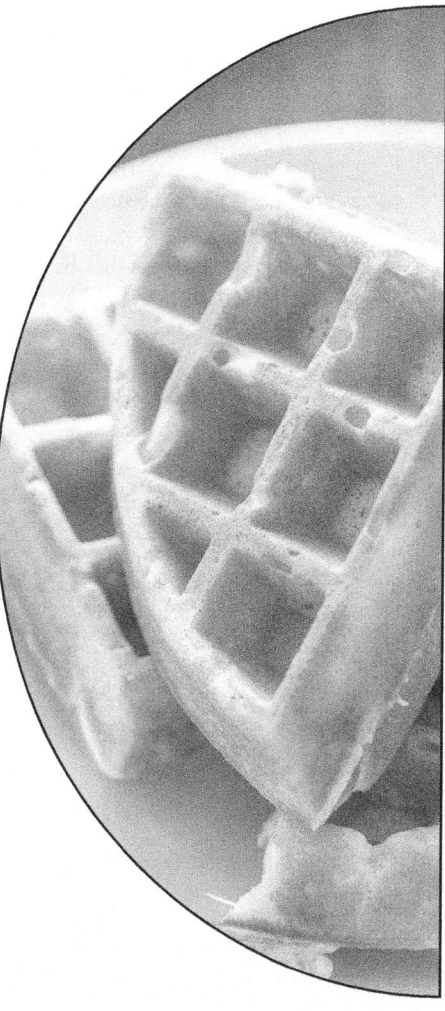

EGG AND BACON BREAKFAST MUFFINS

Preparation Time: 40 minutes
Cooking Time: 25 minutes
Servings: 2

INGREDIENTS

- 4 large eggs
- 4 bacon of slices, cooked and crisped
- 1/3 cup of green onions, chopped green stem only
- Salt and black pepper, to taste
- ¼ teaspoon of paprika

DIRECTIONS

1. Preheat the oven to 350 ºF and lightly grease muffin tin cavities.
2. Whisk the eggs in a bowl and add green onions, bacon, paprika, salt and black pepper.
3. Pour this mixture into the muffin tin cavities and transfer to the oven.
4. Bake for about 25 minutes and remove from oven to serve.

EGG BACON FAT BOMBS

Preparation Time: 15 minutes
Cooking Time: 15 minutes
Servings: 2

INGREDIENTS

- ¼ cup of butter, softened
- 4 large slices of bacon, baked
- 2 large eggs, boiled
- 2 tablespoons of mayonnaise
- Salt and black pepper, to taste

DIRECTIONS

1. Preheat the oven to 375 ºF and lightly grease a baking tray.
2. Put the bacon on the baking tray and bake for about 15 minutes.
3. Remove from the oven, crumble it and set aside.
4. Mash the boiled eggs with butter, mayonnaise, salt and black pepper with a fork.
5. Refrigerate for about 1 hour and then form small balls out of this mixture.
6. Roll the balls into the bacon crumbles and refrigerate for an hour to serve.

NUTRITION

- Calories: 180
- Total Fat: 16.2 g
- Saturated Fat: 7.4 g
- Cholesterol: 98 mg
- Sodium: 406 mg
- Total Carbohydrates: 1.5 g
- Dietary Fiber: 0 g
- Total Sugars: 0.5 g

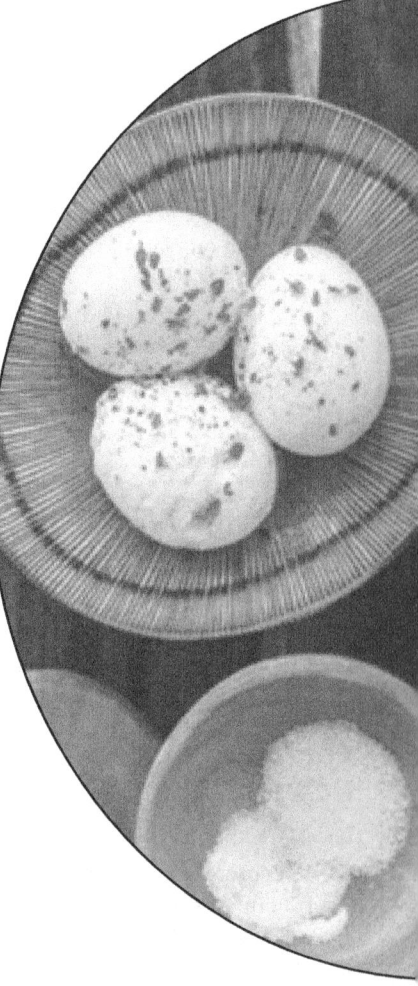

SOFT BOILED EGGS WITH BUTTER AND THYME

Preparation Time: 20 minutes
Cooking Time: 15 minutes
Servings: 2

INGREDIENTS

- 2 tablespoons of butter, melted
- 3 large eggs
- ½ teaspoon of black pepper
- 2 tablespoons of thyme leaves
- ½ teaspoon of Himalayan pink salt

DIRECTIONS

1. Boil the eggs in water for about 6 minutes and then put under cold water.
2. Peel the eggs and dip in the melted butter.
3. Top with thyme leaves and season with salt and black pepper to serve.

NUTRITION

- Calories: 145
- Total Fat: 12.8 g
- Saturated Fat: 6.5 g
- Cholesterol: 206 mg
- Sodium: 631 mg
- Total Carbohydrates: 1.8 g
- Dietary Fiber: 0.8 g
- Total Sugars: 0.4 g
- Protein: 6.6 g

CHAPTER 11.

21 Day Meal Plan

Day	Breakfast	Sides	Dessert
1	Shrimp Skillet	Spinach Rolls	Matcha Crepe Cake
2	Coconut Yogurt with Chia Seeds	Goat Cheese Fold-Overs	Pumpkin Spices Mini Pies
3	Chia Pudding	Crepe Pie	Nut Bars
4	Egg **Fat:** Bombs	Coconut Soup	Pound Cake
5	Morning "Grits"	Fish Tacos	Tortilla Chips with Cinnamon Recipe
6	Scotch Eggs	Cobb Salad	Granola Yogurt with Berries
7	Bacon Sandwich	Cheese Soup	Berry Sorbet
8	Noatmeal	Tuna Tartare	Coconut Berry Smoothie
9	Breakfast Bake with Meat	Clam Chowder	Coconut Milk Banana Smoothie
10	Breakfast Bagel	Asian Beef Salad	Mango Pineapple Smoothie
11	Egg and Vegetable Hash	Keto Carbonara	Raspberry Green Smoothie
12	Cowboy Skillet	Cauliflower Soup with	Loaded Berries Smoothie

13	Feta Quiche	Prosciutto-Wrapped Asparagus	Papaya Banana and Kale Smoothie
14	Bacon Pancakes	Stuffed Bell Peppers	Green Orange Smoothie
15	Waffles	Stuffed Eggplants with Goat Cheese	Double Berries Smoothie
16	Chocolate Shake	Korma Curry	Energizing **Protein:** Bars
17	Eggs in Portobello Mushroom Hats	Zucchini Bars	Sweet and Nutty Brownies
18	Matcha **Fat:** Bombs	Mushroom Soup	Keto Macho Nachos
19	Keto Smoothie Bowl	Stuffed Portobello Mushrooms	Peanut Butter Choco Banana Gelato with Mint
20	Salmon Omelet	Lettuce Salad	Cinnamon Peaches and Yogurt
21	Hash Brown	Onion Soup	Pear Mint Honey Popsicles

CONCLUSION

Thank you for reading the DASH Diet! We hope you have found this book entertaining and, most of all, informative. Remember that good health is a lifelong process and a journey. Don't despair when you slip up on occasion. Just climb back on board! The DASH diet is based on a pyramid, with the most frequently consumed items as the base. That would be fruits and vegetables. These items are supposed to be consumed liberally, in servings of 8-10 per day, with 4-5 servings of vegetables and 4-5 servings of fruits. Next, 6-8 servings of whole grains are to be eaten daily. While 2-3 dairy servings are consumed per day, meat is eaten in relative moderation. Only lean cuts of skinless poultry and fish are eaten regularly in 3-4 ounce portions. Oils are allowed only in tiny amounts and nuts with at most 1 serving per day.

The DASH diet was originally designed to help patients with hypertension manage their blood pressure without using medications. Although it wasn't designed for weight loss, patients found they did lose weight while following the diet. The DASH diet doesn't use calorie counting or any complicated point systems. Instead, food portions are measured, and there are simple rules for daily portions.

This diet program was initially developed in the early 1990s. Back then, ideas about the role of fat in the diet were quite different from today. In those times, it was believed that fat was the cause of heart disease and stroke, and so doctors sought to promote very low-fat diets. However, since that time, doctors have learned the role of fat in the diet is far more complicated than originally believed. In fact, fat, with the exception of a small number of bad fats, is good for health. Furthermore, fat helps dieters refrain from overeating because it leaves you feeling satiated and full of energy.

The Dash Diet Cookbook will have you hacking out your cutlery in no time so you can finally become a healthier human being! It's all about being healthy and learning to enjoy the foods you eat again. We have concluded that Dash Diet Cookbook is an excellent way of losing weight and following a healthy, balanced diet.

If you're ready to get started, the Dash Diet Cookbook is here to help. There's something for everyone in this book, from breakfast items like oatmeal and French toast to dinner side dishes like zucchini noodles and ranch dressing. Feel great about what you eat with the Dash Diet Cookbook!

Consider this work as your guide to the Dash Diet Cookbook. If you have been following the diet for any amount of time, you surely found the information in this guide very informative. Take advantage of the resources provided in each chapter to ensure you succeed on this program and get a much better health.

Dear Reader,
I hope you did enjoy the book and are now closer to your goals. I genuinely hope you are and this book helps you.
Would you be open to leaving a review on Amazon? It's cool if you'd prefer not to, but leaving a review will help me understand what my readers like and what they do not like. I assure you that I read all of the reviews and consider them when writing the next book. Just put down a few words about your thoughts. I will very much appreciate it.
I wish you all the best
Danielle De Mayo

Made in the USA
Monee, IL
06 September 2021